AF814803

WORKING METHODS IN MODERN SCIENCE

EDITED BY PROFESSOR KURT FISCHBECK

AUTORADIOGRAPHY

by

Dipl.-Chem. Dr. H. A. FISCHER
Max-Planck-Institute for Brain Research,
Neurochemical Research Group, Frankfurt/Main, Germany

and

Professor Dipl.-Chem. Dr. G. WERNER
Max-Planck-Institute for Brain Research,
Neurochemical Research Group, Frankfurt/Main, Germany

With 93 figures and 14 tables

W DE G

WALTER DE GRUYTER
Berlin · New York 1971

Translated from an expanded version of the first German edition by Professor M. R. F. Ashworth, Chair of Organic Analysis of the University of the Saar, W. Germany.

The quotation of registered names, trade names, trade marks, etc. in this book does not imply, even in the absence of a specific statement, that such names are exempt from laws and regulations protecting trade marks, etc. and therefore free for general use.

ISBN 3 11 003523 5

Library of Congress Catalog Card Number 70-164842.

©

Copyright 1970 u. 1971 by Walter de Gruyter & Co. Berlin.
All rights reserved, including those of translation into foreign languages. No part of this book may be reproduced in any form — by photoprint, microfilm, or any other means — nor transmitted nor translated into a machine language without written permission from the publisher.
Printed in Germany by Walter de Gruyter & Co., Berlin.
Cover designed by U. Hanisch, Berlin.

FOREWORD TO THE ENGLISH EDITION

This is basically a translation of the 1st German Edition of "Autoradiographie." Mistakes and unclear passages in the original were corrected where found. Some new references have been included to keep the work up to date.
Figures 1, 2, 4, 16, 64, 80, 90, 91, and 93 are reproduced directly from the German Edition, hence commas are to be seen where periods would normally be in English usage.
The authors and publisher are especially grateful to Professor M. R. F. Ashworth of Saarbrücken for the translation. Our thanks also to Dr. E. Schmatolla of Frankfurt for his help in the final reading of the proofs.

Frankfurt am Main and Berlin, Spring 1971

The authors Walter de Gruyter & Co

FOREWORD TO THE GERMAN EDITION

Up to the end of 1969, some 10,000 publications had appeared which were concerned with autoradiography: This method has applications in many scientific subjects but, apart from a few summarising treatments*, no inclusive presentation exists so far which can be regarded unequivocally as an introduction to the practical and theoretical fundamentals of this extensive domain.
We planned originally to publish a type of handbook, aimed at giving those interested rapid guidance in the methods and results of autoradiographic investigations. Limitations were, however, imposed on us in this connection. We have had likewise to abandon a complete bibliography to the present monograph. As far as possible, we have cited the newer publications in order to facilitate access to the original literature. We hope that the book will close a noticeable information gap.
We have striven constantly to provide a guide which, firstly, will introduce the fundamentals, methods and problems of autoradiography to the reader who is interested, yet without experience in practical details; and which will, through numerous tips, help him to save time, expense and effort. Secondly, we wanted to give information on those problems which can at present be attacked with greater or lesser success by autoradiographic methods.

---

* See Section 9.2

The book is accordingly divided into several sections. Since the application of autoradiographic methods extends over a wide range of subjects, a fairly mixed reading public is to be expected and a brief initial section is devoted to information about the phenomenon of radioactivity, radioactive isotopes and labelling; this part (Chapters 2. & 3.) is intended only for the less scientifically equipped reader. In the next sections, *autoradiographic methods for macroscopic, light-microscopic* and *electron-microscopic specimens* are treated in detail; the practical side is explained and discussed in each case with the help of examples. Special aids are discussed here regarding production of autoradiograms and also of the preparations themselves (at least as far as they are concerned with autoradiography). Necessary theoretical considerations and illustrations of the limitations of the methods, of resolving power and of the photographic process and related effects are included; this yields an inclusive presentation of the whole autoradiographic domain. A final section is devoted to the basic principles and methods of *quantitative autoradiography*. Only a few typical examples of application amongst the huge number of publications in the autoradiographic sphere could be chosen for illustrating the efficiency of the method; in particular, those investigations were picked which the reader without specialist knowledge could understand. It is unnecessary to mention that this selection implies no valuation.

The book is written from practical experience for practical use. The authors and publishers are grateful for hints, suggestions for improvement and wishes which may be able to receive consideration in a new edition or translation. They thank especially for their kindness in providing manuscripts and diagrams: Dr. BRIGITTE SCHULTZE of Würzburg; Professor L. DESCARRIES of Paris; Professor W. HERRMANN of Leipzig; Professor W. MAURER of Würzburg; Dr. H. P. ROHR of Basel; Professor A. W. ROGERS of Birmingham; Professor E. STÖCKER of Würzburg; and Professor S. ULLBERG of Stockholm.

We should like to thank especially our assistant Fräulein SIGRID THEL for her valuable help in all preliminary work necessary for preparing the manuscript. We should like to thank Dr. HUBERT KORR for reading the proofs. Not least we wish to thank also the publishers Walter de Gruyter & Co.

Frankfurt am Main, Spring 1970 H. A. FISCHER G. WERNER

CONTENTS

1. INTRODUCTION

Photographic emulsions can be converted into a developable state through high-energy photons, such as light or X-rays, or by interaction with α-radiation, electrons and other high-energy particles which, for example, arise during atomic transmutation processes. This property led BECQUEREL in 1896 to the discovery of radioactive radiation. For a long time after that, photographic plates were used to detect radiation yielded during atomic transmutations. This method was later replaced by more sensitive physical measuring procedures. Recently, however, photosensitive plates have regained significance in this connection in atomic physics where they are employed to detect and identify products of nuclear fission and disintegration. Photographic emulsions are used also in dosimeters; these, in the form of pocket badges, are legally obligatory for surveillance or control of persons exposed to radiation danger. Autoradiography is a further field in which photographic emulsions are finding increased and important use.

If a photographic emulsion is exposed for a time in the immediate neighbourhood of a radioactive preparation and subsequently developed, a blackened picture is obtained under certain conditions. This *autoradiogram* is related closely to the frequency of occurrence and distribution of the radioactive atoms in the preparation. *Autoradiography* is the term for this use of photographic emulsions to study occurrence and distribution of radioactive substances. Autoradiography has a wide range of uses. So far, easily the largest number of pertinent publications has concerned medical and biological research; autoradiography has, however, been applied also to solve special problems in geology, meteorology, solid state physics, chemical analysis, criminology and pest control, to name only a few other fields. Since the spheres and objects of application and the problems posed are so diverse, many variations of method have been described.

The nomenclature in the literature is not uniform. We therefore consider that "*autoradiography*" ought to refer only to the *method* and *not* to the resulting picture, as is often the case in publications in German. The picture should be termed an "*autoradiogram.*" It would be idle to discuss here all the synonyms employed for the method, the more so because they are gradually being replaced by the terms used here. A few roughly equivalent expressions for autoradiography are: autography, autophotography, curiegraphy and radiography. Our nomenclature accords with that proposed by TAUXE, MOSER and BOYD [439] with one difference: based on PREUSS and JOFTES [353] we have extended the term autoradiography to cover methods using photographic emulsions for detection of the distribution of radioactive materials *on* the surface of specimens as well as *in* them. We feel that this definition is more sensible since it eliminates the arbitrary and unjustified distinction between inner and peripheral occurrence of radioactive substance in the material studied. It then includes also histological applications ("*histoautoradiography*") and all other uses of autoradiography.

A comment must be made also on our terms "*macroscopic*," "*microscopic*" and "*electron-microscopic*." Under "*macroscopic*" specimens we mean those, the autoradiograms of which can be evaluated without the help of any microscope technique, i. e., without any particular optical magnification. Usually it involves mere detection of radioactive substances on the surfaces of larger samples, such as minerals, paper- and thin layer chromatograms, electropherograms or on sections of other larger specimens (e. g. "*whole-body autoradiography*"). "*Microscopic autoradiography*" is linguistically inaccurate and ought really to be replaced by "autoradiography of microscopic specimens." It concerns the preparation of autoradiograms, the evaluation of which requires light-microscopic magnification. All specimens where evaluation demands still higher resolution than that of the light microscope are referred to as "*electron-microscopic*". There are still considerable difficulties of method associated with this last named autoradiographic technique and results are accordingly rather unsatisfactory. A larger number of relevant publications has nevertheless appeared.

2. PHYSICAL BASES OF RADIOACTIVITY

Radioactive atoms are distinguished from one another through: the maximum energy liberated on disintegration (decay); the nature of the disintegration products; and the time interval during which, e. g. half of a number of identical atomic nuclei radioactively disintegrates. The number of disintegrations per unit time is directly proportional to the amount of starting material capable of disintegration. Thus, for instance, the number of changes from tritium ^3_1H to helium ^3_2He is directly proportional to the amount of tritium. The *law of radioactive disintegration* follows from this; it states that

$$N_t = N_0 \cdot e^{-\lambda t}$$

where N_0 = number of atoms present at time t_0
N_t = number of atoms still present after time t.
e = 2.71828....

Each radioactive isotope has its characteristic λ, the so-called *disintegration constant* (radioactive constant, decay constant). The greater this value is, the swifter the decay. The *half-life* τ gives a clearer picture of the tendency of an isotope to decay than does the disintegration constant. This is the time during which one half of the atoms originally present disintegrate. Tritium, for example, has a half-life of 12.26 years. Half-life and disintegration constant are related:

$$\tau = \frac{0.693}{\lambda}.$$

The various radioactive isotopes have widely differing half-lives. These range from fractions of a second to several million years. Only those isotopes with half-lives of at least a few days can be considered for autoradiography (cf Section 7.5.).
The concept of *average life period* is sometimes used for radioactive substances. This is the time during which any original amount is reduced to the fraction $\frac{1}{e}$, i. e., ca $37^0/_0$. Disintegration constant, half-life and average life period of radioactive isotopes are characteristic natural constants which cannot be influenced by any chemical or physical means whatever.
Radioisotopes rarely occur "pure." Concentrates of a radioactive isotope in a mixture are, however, often available. A unit of radioactivity of a substance has been agreed on for all these cases; it is the number of disintegrations taking place in unit time in the particular substance. This unit is called the *Curie* (*C*). In a substance of activity 1 *C*, $3.70 \cdot 10^{10}$ disintegrations occur per second.

The curie is a measure only of the radioactivity of substances and not of the danger which handling these substances may mean. The radiation dangers to life of a substance depend on many factors, notably, its activity, the energy liberated during the decay process, the nature of the radiation and the proximity. This danger is measured as radiation dosage in röntgen units (*r*).
In practice, not only the radioactivity of a substance is of interest but also the concentration of this activity. The concept of *specific activity* was consequently introduced. With substances of unknown or inhomogeneous chemical composition, this specific activity is based on mass, having thus the dimensions of curie/gram. The unit curie/mole or curie/val* is often employed since the mole rather than the physical unit of mass is more useful chemically. A mole of substance always contains the same number of molecules, $6.023 \cdot 10^{23}$.
One can easily see that the specific activity has an upper limit, attained when the particular isotopes or radioactively labelled molecules are not diluted by inactive material. These theoretical upper limits are given in Table 1 for some frequently used radioisotopes.

Table 1
Maximum specific activities at 100% isotope concentration

Isotope	Half life	C/mVal	C/mg
^{36}Cl	ca $3 \cdot 10^5$ a	$1.1 \cdot 10^{-3}$	$0.3 \cdot 10^{-3}$
^{14}C	5760 a	$6.2 \cdot 10^{-2}$	$4.4 \cdot 10^{-3}$
^{3}H	12.26 a	29	9.6
^{35}S	87 d	$1.488 \cdot 10^3$	42.8
^{32}P	14.3 d	$9.12 \cdot 10^3$	285
^{131}I	8.05 d	$16.1 \cdot 10^3$	123

The energy liberated during radioactive disintegration can be emitted as radiation in various ways, e. g., as α- or β-particles or as γ-quanta. α-Emission is shown almost only by elements of atomic number over 82, i. e., those naturally radioactive. α-Particles are helium nuclei and possess two protons and two neutrons. A nucleus suffering such a radioactive decay therefore loses this charge and mass. For example, radium (atomic number 88) yields "radium emanation," an inert gas with the element name radon (atomic number 86):

$$^{226}_{88}\mathrm{Ra} \longrightarrow {}^{222}_{86}\mathrm{Rn} + {}^{4}_{2}\mathrm{He}\,.$$

β-Emission may be of electrons or of their electrical opposite numbers, *positrons*. A neutron is converted into a proton by β-emission. A new

* 1 gram equivalent (1 val) is also termed 1 Tom nowadays.

nucleus is produced of the same mass number (*isobaric*) but of atomic number one unit larger, e. g.,

$$^{32}_{15}P \longrightarrow ^{32}_{16}S + \beta^- .$$

When a positron is emitted, a proton is transformed into a neutron and the atomic number of the resulting nucleus is one unit less than that of the disintegrating nucleus. Positron-emitters are rare and insignificant for autoradiography. β^+-Particles of high energy are indistinguishable from equivalent electrons in their action on photographic emulsions. β^+-Radiation does not occur externally below a certain particle energy because positrons and electrons then unite with emission of a γ-quantum.

β-Emitters are often *γ-emitters* also. γ-Radiation is electrically neutral. γ-Quanta are photons in the X-ray region of the electromagnetic spectrum. They arise when an initially unstable nucleus results from the radioactive decay. It is stabilised from its "excited" state by emission of γ-rays. (Fig. 1).

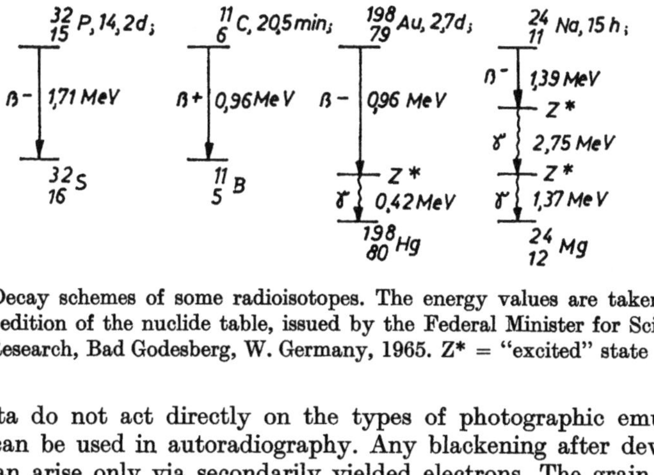

Fig. 1. Decay schemes of some radioisotopes. The energy values are taken from the 2nd edition of the nuclide table, issued by the Federal Minister for Scientific Research, Bad Godesberg, W. Germany, 1965. Z* = "excited" state

γ-Quanta do not act directly on the types of photographic emulsion which can be used in autoradiography. Any blackening after development can arise only via secondarily yielded electrons. The grain yield (Section 5.2.4.) is minute in relation to the γ-quanta emitted. Yet, although γ-radiation is of no significance for autoradiographic practice, the action of the radiation must not be disregarded. Its danger to the experimenter due to the extensive radiation range in vacuum and the powerful penetration of material must be allowed for.

α- and β-Particles in particular are important in autoradiographic practice. α-Particles from the same isotope are always emitted with the same energy. β-Particles, however, possess only certain energies which vary continuously between zero and a maximum. The *maximum energy* is given always as a characteristic for a β-emitter. Since a distribution

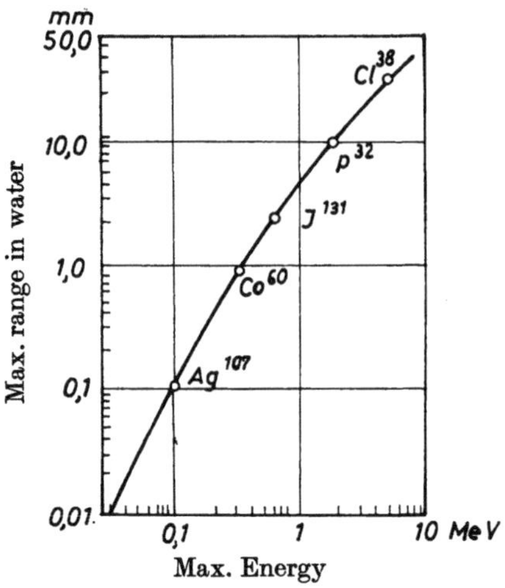

Fig. 2. Dependence of range of electron emission on energy in the 0.01—10 MeV region. Medium: water. The isotopes are drawn in according to their maximum energies. Modified according to GLEASON, TAYLOR and TABERN [157]

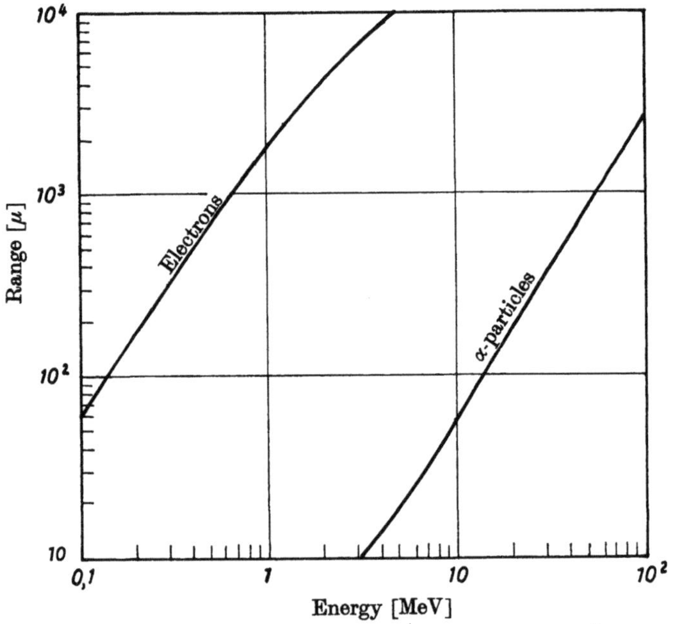

Fig. 3. Relation between energy and range for fine grained Kodak nuclear track emulsions. From [234]

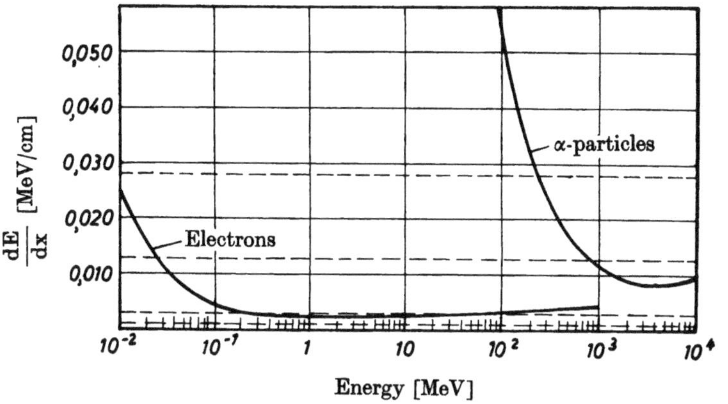

Fig. 4. Dependence of energy loss on the individual energy during passage of α- or β-radiation through air. From [234]

of range attained results from the energy distribution of an emitter, the energy is an important magnitude in autoradiography, e. g., in connection with the realisable resolution (Section 6.2.). The range of a β-particle always exceeds that of an α-particle of the same energy. This can be explained through the differing masses and particle sizes. Their small mass means that β-particles are highly scattered by contact with matter. The paths are therefore not linear. Energy is lost in ionising the penetrated medium. The ionisation density is far smaller for β-particles than for α-particles. The ionisation density or energy lost per unit length of path covered is a function of the energy. The density of the medium plays a part also. Figures 2, 3 and 4 show the relation between energy and range for a medium of density unity (e. g., water or, roughly, organic tissue) and for nuclear track emulsions; and also the relation between energy and energy loss for electrons and α-particles (cf also Fig. 58). The curves in Fig. 4 possess a minimum, corresponding to the lowest ionisation power. The minimum for β-ionisation is at about 1 MeV. This value applies to all media, including photographic emulsions. It is worthy of notice since many β-emitters suitable for autoradiography have energies in this region. They act less on photographic emulsions than do those from emitters of lower energy.

The superior ionising power of α-radiation, as evident from Fig. 4, explains also the higher sensitivity of detection in α-track autoradiography (Section 7.2.).

3. LABELLING WITH RADIOACTIVE ISOTOPES

By *labelling* (*tagging*) in the present context is understood the substitution of one or several atoms in molecules or other combinations of atoms by their radioactive isotopes. This labelling is the only possible way of following the fate of a particular atom during chemical reactions, such as in metabolic processes. Since labelled material is always used in autoradiography, we wish to describe types and possibilities of labelling in the following pages.

Molecules can be tagged in various ways. Thus, e. g., radiocarbon ($^{14}_{6}C$) or hydrogen (tritium, $^{3}_{1}H$) may be introduced into the molecules of organic compounds. One distinguishes between *specific* and *non-specific* labelling. In the former, a definite atom is replaced, the position of which in the molecule is known; e. g., the C-atom in a methyl group. *Specific* labelling requires deliberate syntheses which are now and then complex and tedious. A "simple" exchange of an atom within a molecule by an isotope is not possible on a reasonable preparative scale, except for hydrogen. Starting material is used in which the isotope to be introduced is already present; or one begins with the elements themselves in which the natural isotopic distribution has already been modified in favour of the desired tracer isotope.

Non-specifically labelled compounds suffice for many purposes. The position of the tracer isotope is not fixed and can vary from molecule to molecule. The desired molecule must generally be synthesised in non-specific labelling also. This can be circumvented only in the case of tritium. Hydrogen-containing compounds which are maintained long enough in a tritium-containing atmosphere exchange their hydrogen for the heavy isotope via reaction processes that are not yet fully understood. The energy liberated during decay of the tritium ($E = 0.018$ MeV) plays a decisive rôle in the reaction. This *Wilzbach-synthesis** has several modifications. The chance of replacement by tritium is not identical for all hydrogen atoms in a molecule. In some cases, admittedly few, the Wilzbach method thus labels compounds largely specifically.

Radiochemicals prepared by the Wilzbach method or biologically are termed in the English and German language literature as labelled uniformly (uniform), non-specifically (unspezifisch) or also statistically (statistisch). Yet it is certainly not uniform labelling and the labelling is non-specific only with respect to the site in the molecule. The distribution of activity over the atoms in different parts of the molecule is

* A monograph on preparation, measurement and use of ^{3}H-labelled compounds via WILZBACH, written by M. WENZEL and P. E. SCHULZE, was published by Walter de Gruyter & Co. in 1962.

not uniform. The suggestion has been made of calling such substances polytopic-inhomogeneously labelled and to distinguish them from the polytopic-homogeneously labelled compounds. Depending on whether one or more atoms of the same atomic number in a molecule have been replaced by isotopes, one should refer to monotopic-, ditopic-, tritopic-labelled compounds, etc. When radioactive isotopes of various atomic numbers are introduced into a molecule, the substances are spoken of as heterogeneously labelled [398]. One refers to heterotopic-labelled compounds when they differ from one another through having had isotopes incorporated into different sites in the molecule.

A disadvantage of the Wilzbach method is that, in addition to the labelling, numerous chemical bonds in the molecule may be broken and reform anew. By-products thus always appear which may possess high specific activities and which must be separated. The great advantage of the method is that it permits radioactive compounds to be obtained which can be prepared through chemical synthesis only with difficulty or not at all if their structure is inadequately known (e. g., natural products). It has been possible to label successfully even viruses in this way.

Other ways of labelling which can be important for autoradiography are: surface adsorption of radioactive reagents (Section 4.1.1.); ion adsorption (Section 4.4.4.); employment of a chemical homologue (Section 4.1.1.); and neutron activation (Section 4.1.1. amongst others). Examples are treated in the relevant section.

Radiation resulting from decay of radioactive isotopes is detected through its action on unexposed photographic plates. Further information about the chemical bonds in the emitter cannot be obtained autoradiographically. For example, it is not possible to distinguish between radioactive sulphur present as sulphate or in a thiol group.

Reference may be made in conclusion to a danger which can occur through chemical changes of the labelled substances added to the specimen under examination for interpreting the autoradiograms. On no account should the blackened picture be taken as giving the distribution pattern of the originally applied labelled compound without having tested to what extent this pattern is due to radiation from possible reaction products of the radioactive starting substance which also contain the *tracer* atom. This can apply particularly to autoradiograms of biological specimens on account of the multitude of possible metabolites (cf Section 4.3.6.).

Further, an unexpected exchange of tritium with ordinary hydrogen may take place in organic molecules during metabolism, although the labelled starting material displays no labile bonds during incubation with acids or bases [175].

Many labelled organic compounds are commercially available, especially known products of metabolism or those of particular pharmacological interest.

4. AUTORADIOGRAPHY OF MACROSCOPIC SPECIMENS

This chapter contains applications of the autoradiographic technique to specimens where observation and evaluation require as a rule no microscope or only slight magnification. Examples, as typical as possible, are chosen from various specialist fields. Primarily, details are given about the autoradiographic technique. A discussion of the merits and possibilities of application of autoradiography has been preferred to a presentation of specialist problem formulations.

4.1. Investigations of metals and alloys

4.1.1. General information about metal autoradiography

Autoradiography is a valuable supplement to many testing and analysis procedures employed in metallurgy, material testing and corrosion research. This applies especially to detection of traces on surface and interface layers only a few molecules thick. In addition, processes in homogeneous phase which would evade any chemical analysis can be observed autoradiographically. Examples are self-diffusion in metals or mutual interpenetration of neighbouring metals, such as in electronic construction elements or bimetallic devices [159; 372].
Practically only lead and bismuth isotopes, from the natural decay series, were available to Tammann and Bandel in 1933 when they introduced autoradiography into metallography. After having been added to alloys of lead and bismuth, these radioisotopes gave surprisingly well-defined autoradiographic pictures of the structure. The simple contact autoradiographic procedure of that time is capable nowadays of extensive improvement by employing suitable types of emulsion [308; 160; 209; 140; 129; 4; 25; 237].
Glawitsch gives hints for preparing autoradiograms of metallic materials, such as sintered products, partly melted material or metallic impregnations; this was in connection with autoradiographic studies of the silver-gold system which consisted of a continuous series of mixed crystals [156]. Samples for autoradiographic investigation, of about 4 mm cross-section, were embedded in a fusible resin, such as polyester, or also in Wood's alloy, and polished. The activity was quoted which was necessary for a sample to yield autoradiograms 24 hours later with measurable blackening; e. g., for ^{110}Ag and *Kodak*

Autoradiographic Plates, it was about 12 µC. It had to be borne in mind that the photographic emulsion suffers blackening as a result of chemography through contact with the Wood's alloy (Section 4.1.2.). This chemography could be prevented by thin, hydrophobic films of formvar, prepared from a 0.5% solution of polyvinyl formal in chloroform; the resolution suffered no recognisable loss as a result. *Kodak Autoradiographic Plates* are universally recommended in metal autoradiography because they yield pictures with clearest contrast and minimum background (Fig. 5). This film is used as in the stripping film technique, described fully in Section 5.2.
Direct labelling of individual alloy components by adding suitable radioactive isotopes to the metal melt is not always possible, e. g., for reasons of protection against radiation. *Neutron activation* is a useful supplementary technique and substitute for direct labelling. The metal samples under study are then exposed to a neutron source of high flux density; mainly so-called (n, γ)-processes then take place, i. e., emission of γ-quanta accompanying neutron capture. Many nuclides are thus transformed into heavier isotopes which are frequently β-emitters. Neutron activation is especially suitable for metallic samples since they

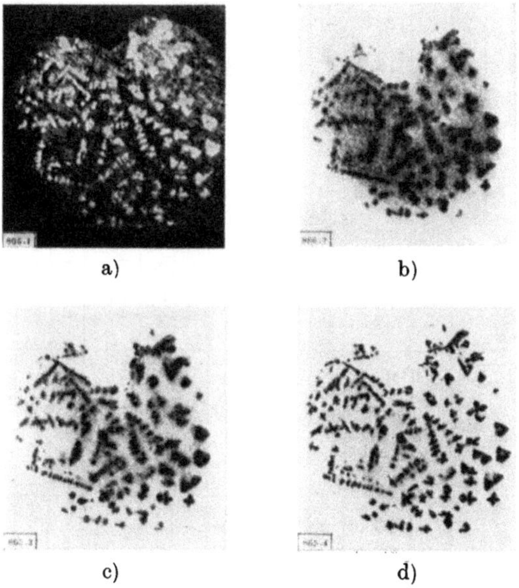

Fig. 5. Comparison of autoradiograms of a ^{110}Ag-Bi alloy, various film materials. From [156]

a) HNO_3-etching of the alloy; b) Contact autoradiogram with *Kodak Dental X-ray Film*; c) Contact autoradiogram with *Perutz Perulith Thin-Layer Film*; d) Stripping film autoradiogram using *Kodak Autoradiographic Plate*

Table 2

Data on some metals for activation through (n, γ)-processes, after RADWAN [358]. The values are based on a neutron source of medium power (flow density of 10^{11} neutrons/sec/cm^2). Which specimen component becomes labelled in reasonable amounts can be estimated from the increase in activity with the time of irradiation and the subsequent fall in activity

Starting isotope	% Present in natural isotope mixture	Isotope formed through n, γ-process	Half-life T	Activities after various irradiation times					Saturation activity (μc/g)	Saturation time
				0.1 h	1 h	10 h	100 h	500 h		
^{23}Na	100	^{24}Na	14.97 h	180	1,626	13,356	35,640	36,000	36,000	150 h
^{27}Al	100	^{28}Al	2.27 min	10,580	12,600	12,600	12,600	12,600	12,600	22.7 min
^{31}P	· 100	^{32}P	14.22 d	1.83	20	200	1,800	6,800	10,000	142.2 d
^{34}S	4.215	^{35}S	87.1 d	—	0.17	1.8	18.1	90.7	520	871 d
^{44}Ca	2.06	^{45}Ca	164 d	—	0.095	0.96	9.5	47.7	508	1640 d
^{50}Cr	4.31	^{51}Cr	27.8 d	1.87	18.8	188.2	1,882	7,330	18,100	278 d
^{55}Mn	100	^{56}Mn	2.58 h	10,360	92,700	366,200	394,000	394,000	394,000	25.8 h
^{54}Fe	5.84	^{55}Fe	2.6 a	—	0.127	1.275	12,75	63.75	4,250	26 a
^{58}Fe	0.31	^{59}Fe	45.1 d	—	0.051	0.512	5,12	25.6	87	451 d
^{59}Co	100	^{60m}Co	10.47 min 5.24 a	1.4	14	140	1,386	6,730	990,000	52.4 a
^{64}Ni	1.16	^{65}Ni	2.564 h	12.4	111	438	470	470	470	25.64 h
^{63}Cu	69.1	^{64}Cu	12.8 h	416	4,100	32,000	75,500	76,000	76,000	128 h
^{64}Zn	48.89	^{65}Zn	245 d	0.066	0.63	6.31	63.1	315.6	5,450	2450 d
^{68}Zn	18.56	^{69m}Zn	13.8 h	2.15	21.1	164	420	430	430	138 h
		^{69}Zn	57 min	310	2,288	4,426	4,426	4,426	4,426	9.5 h
^{70}Ge	20.55	^{70}Ge	11.4 d	5.6	50	457	4,100	12,900	18,300	114 d
^{75}As	100	^{76}As	26.4 h	300	3,030	26,106	105,560	114,000	114,000	264 h

Table 2 (continued)

Starting isotope	% Present in natural isotope mixture	Isotope formed through n, γ-process	Half-life T	Activities after various irradiation times					Saturation activity	Saturation time
				0.1 h	1 h	10 h	100 h	500 h	(μc/g)	
^{89}Y	100	^{90}Y	64.2 h	28.7	256	4,520	15,400	22,300	23,300	642 h
^{98}Mo	23.75	^{99}Mo	66 h	1.87	18.4	183.7	1,137	1,700	1,750	660 h
^{109}Ag	48.65	^{110m}Ag	253 d	0.32	3	28	265	1,300	23,130	2530 d
^{114}Cd	28.86	^{115m}Cd	43 d	—	—	3.84	40	163	575	430 d
^{114}Cd	28.86	^{115}Cd	53 h	14.4	100	600	3,300	4,500	4,520	530 h
^{112}Sn	0.95	^{113}Sn	119 d	—	0.04	0.3936	3.936	19,68	164	1190 d
^{120}Sn	32.97	^{121}Sn	27.5 h	0.81	9.66	89.6	497	640	640	275 h
^{121}Sb	57.25	^{122}Sb	2.8 d	46	536	5,356	33,440	51,690	52,000	28 d
^{123}Sb	42.75	^{124}Sb	60.9 d	0.66	6.58	65.8	658	3,290	14,000	609 d
^{184}W	30.6	^{185}W	75.8 d	0.23	2.17	21.66	217	1,083	5,700	758 d
^{186}W	28.4	^{187}W	24 h	264	2,543	22,180	8,307	88,000	88,000	240 h
^{191}Ir	38.5	^{192}Ir	74.37 d	90	900	8,600	86,200	430,900	228,000	743.7 d
^{193}Ir	61.5	^{194}Ir	19 h	2,450	24,400	202,300	651,900	637	673,000	190 h
^{196}Pt	25.4	^{197}Pt	18 h	5,2	60	500	1,600	1,670	1,670	180 h
^{198}Pt	7.2	^{199}Pt	31 min	300	1,700	2,300	2,300	2,300	2,300	5.2 h
^{197}Au	100	^{198}Au	2.697 d	770	843.7	80,375	519,820	785,300	790,000	26.97 d
^{202}Hg	29.8	^{203}Hg	46.9 d	0.62	6	56,5	550	2,423	9,140	469 d
^{209}Bi	100	^{210}Bi	5,013 d	78	800	8,200	64,770	139,000	147,500	50.13 d

rarely suffer morphological or structural changes in contrast to histological preparations. Some interesting data in this connection are given in Table 2, taken from work of RADWAN [358].

In conclusion, the successful labelling procedure of RABINOWICZ [356] may be referred to. It depends on labelling through surface adsorption of radioactive reagents. Differing labelling patterns may be obtained possibly even through differences alone in the contact potentials of the individual phases. These permit visualisation of inhomogeneities on the surface of the body being investigated which could not be detected at all in an ordinary metallographic study. In this method, the polished, even, metal surface is wetted briefly (seconds suffice) with a solution containing some radioactively labelled reagent which reacts with at least *one* alloy constituent or is adsorbed in traces. For example, if a copper-containing material is briefly immersed in a solution of amyl iodide containing ^{131}I (say 1.5 mC/g), the treated surface then cleaned with suitable solvents and the sample autoradiographed in a plane cutting the treated surface, iodine can be detected autoradiographically which has penetrated along the line of intersection to a depth of 150 atom layers. The depth of penetration can thus be measured or at least estimated autoradiographically. This offers a new possibility of research on the physical and chemical properties of metal surfaces which often play a significant part in catalytic processes.

4.1.2. Artefacts in metal autoradiography

Chemographically induced artefacts have to be reckoned with to a considerable degree in metal autoradiography. Some remarks are thus justified about this usually extremely undesirable phenomenon, the origin of which is difficult to interpret.

As is known, energy is needed to convert a halide crystal into a state capable of photographic development. This energy does not necessarily have to be provided in the form of photons, i. e., electromagnetic radiation; autoradiography owes its existence to this, in fact. Thermal energy also, as the ubiquitous kinetic energy of the molecules ("thermal motion") can lead to formation of photographically developable crystals. Thermal motion and cosmic radiation are the principal causes of increase in the so-called *background* value of photographic emulsions with increasing storage times.

Attention has been drawn to other reasons for photographic blackening in autoradiography which cannot be due to radiation. These effects, termed *chemography*, are difficult to explain. Thus GLAWITSCH [156] reports that direct contact with base metals causes latent blackening of photoemulsions. An explanation may be reduction of the silver ion by metal, or, in the case of alloys, even via local elements. Against this hypothesis must be set the phenomenon discovered by MOSER [312]

in 1842 which has become known as the *Russel effect*; this more general phenomenon is the ability of fresh, newly-formed metal surfaces to "expose" photographic emulsions [389]. Energy-furnishing changes thus occur evidently on newly-prepared metal surfaces. Phenomena of this kind have been known for some time, e. g., triboluminescence with crystals. This is the appearance of light when crystals are pulverised. It is doubtful, however, whether fresh metal surfaces really luminesce. Some authors, such as GRUNBERG [168] are of the opinion that electrons (*exoelectrons*) are emitted from fresh metal surfaces and that these lead to formation of H_2O_2 which in turn yields a latent image.
It is important in practice to know of such sources of error so as to be able to eliminate them if possible, e. g., by coating the surfaces with thin plastic varnish. In order to allow for chemographic effects, one should always carry out a blank experiment in the absence of radioactive substances with every type of specimen to be investigated and under the same conditions as those to be subsequently used. This often yields a "pseudoautoradiogram" and one speaks of *positive chemography.*
An impressive example of such a pseudoautoradiogram can be taken from GROSSKREUTZ [167]. He submitted flat strips of polycrystalline purest aluminium to strain through push-pull. This led to fatigue fractures. Immediately after this treatment, the aluminium samples were coated with stripping film (Section 5.2.) under water and exclusion of daylight, dried at room temperature and exposed for 18 hours. The film was developed, separated from the metal under water, picked up on microscope slides and dried. The film showed blackening like in an autoradiogram, although the particular material contained no radioactive substance (Fig. 6). Blackening was most intense at those places where the material had suffered structural modifications. The pseudoautoradiogram is thus a sensitive means of detecting fatigue fractures in

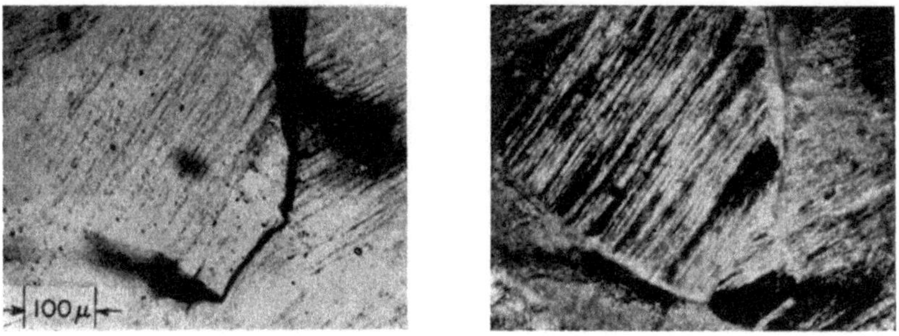

a) b)

Fig. 6

a) Pseudoautoradiogram, yielded through fatigue fractures in aluminium;
b) Same preparation in dark field

From GROSSKREUTZ [167]. See text for details

aluminium; they can be located earlier and more precisely in this way than in the metal microscope. Chemography, otherwise undesirable, can be utilised in this case through the pseudoautoradiographic effect for early diagnosis of fatigue fractures of a metal.
Chemographic effects can be averted only by eliminating all direct contact between the specimen studied and the film material, i. e., by inserting an inert layer [373]. In practice, this layer is prepared in one of several ways: The surface to be studied is coated with a thin foil of plastic; or it is sprayed with a polymer which sets to a cohesive, uniformly thick film. A third way may be mentioned for the sake of completeness. It can be applied to, above all, smaller specimens, as used in electron microscopy; the relevant surfaces of the preparation are subjected to vapour deposition with carbon. Various equipments are commercially available for this purpose, e. g., the high vacuum vaporisation apparatus Micro-BA 3 of the firm *Balzers AG*, Liechtenstein. The value of carbon vapour deposition is still contested. All means serving to hinder contact between the film material and the specimen under investigation act unfavourably on the resolution of the autoradiographic image, at least with low-energy β-radiation. Moreover, the time of exposure may be appreciably lengthened.

4.1.3. Topographical detection of hydrogen in metals

Metallurgical investigations of the penetration of gases, especially hydrogen, into metals and alloys furnish impressive examples of the application of autoradiography. Even at room temperature, appreciable amounts of hydrogen dissolve in many metals, e. g., those of the eighth subgroup of the periodic table. By labelling with tritium it has been possible in some cases to obtain qualitative information about the uptake and transport processes and the storage regions and even quantitative data, e. g., on the rate of diffusion of the tritium. Thus Foster, Gillespie, Jack and Hill [141] studied the occurrence of hydrogen in aluminium; Shiraishi and Nagasaki [409], the behaviour of hydrogen in aluminium-lithium alloys; Erickson and Hardie [124], the localisation of hydrogen inclusions in a zirconium-niobium alloy; and Cupp and Flubacher [88], the diffusion of hydrogen in zirconium and other metals.
We should like to go into a little more detail here about this last-named publication because it seems to us important for autoradiographic practice and because its experimental side is worthy of mention.
The metal sample was charged with hydrogen with the help of the electrolytic cell in Fig. 7. The cathode consisted of the metal sample under investigation. The area of the cathode facing the anode was 4 × 23 mm and the space between the electrodes, 2 mm. A 0.02 N sulphuric acid solution with a specific activity of 100 mC tritium/ml

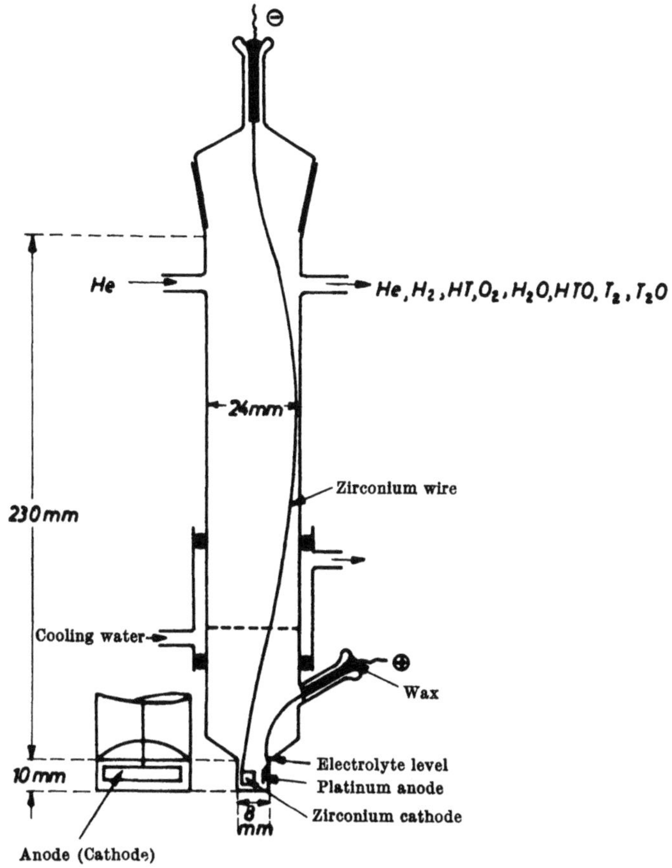

Fig. 7. Diagram with some details of a metal tritiation cell according to CUPP and FLUBACHER [88]

served as electrolyte. About 0.8 ml of electrolyte was decomposed during the 20-hour electrolysis. 0.15% of the hydrogen generated had to remain in the cathode. A temperature of about 80° was attained during electrolysis. After electrolysis, the cathode was cut into 6 pieces, perpendicularly to the hydrogenated surface. Each piece was separately subjected to various temperatures for various periods of time. This treatment caused the tritium gas, concentrated on the surface, to diffuse relatively rapidly into the metal. For the autoradiography, the samples were embedded in a cold-setting plastic (VYNS = *vinylite plastic*) so that only the surface to be studied remained free (Fig. 8).
The authors used *Kodak Autoradiographic Permeable Base Safety Stripping Film* (*Experimental*) as film, on which zirconium and its alloys are

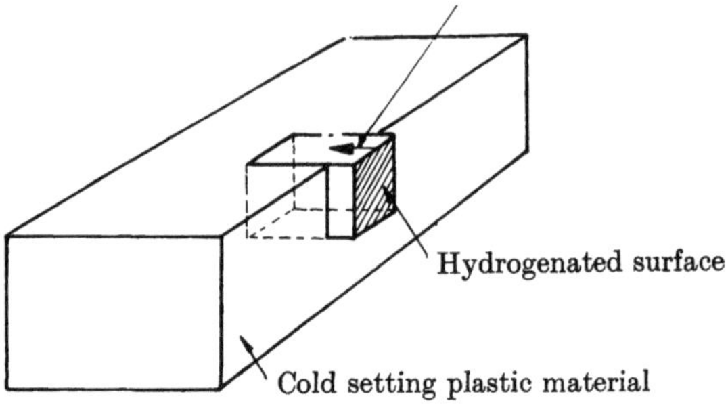

Fig. 8. Embedding a hydrogenated metal sample in a cold-setting plastic for autoradiography. According to CUPP and FLUBACHER [88]

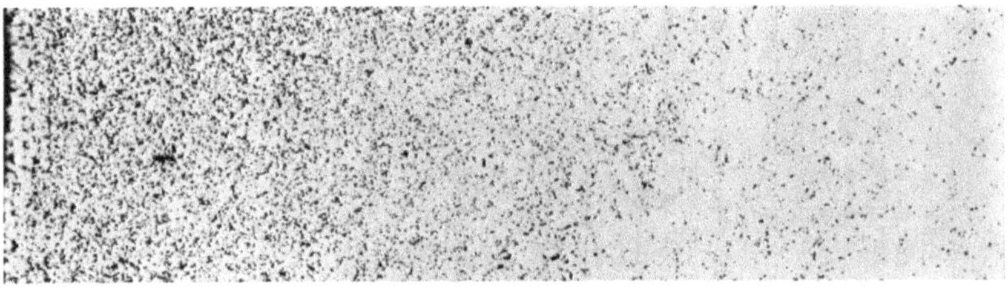

Fig. 9. Autoradiogram of a metal sample, superficially treated with tritium (highly magnified). A concentration profile is formed through heating (252 sec at 240° C) which is clearly recognisable from the blackening. From [88]

claimed not to act chemographically. Times of exposure ranged from 3 hours to 3 days, depending on the sample. Dektol-water (1+1) was used as developer with 1 min developing time. Fixing was performed in *Kodak Acid Fixer*. The autoradiograms were separated from the preparation before the photographic treatment and picked up on microscope slides. They were evaluated with the help of a projection microscope. According to the authors, tritium concentrations of 0.005 ppm still yielded good autoradiograms.

4.1.4. Corrosion phenomena on metals

Work on the oxidation of beryllium through carbon dioxide is the example of autoradiographic investigation in the sphere of metal corrosion which we have chosen. This theme is of special interest since beryllium metal, a good neutron moderator, can be used as a fuel-cladding material in CO_2-cooled reactors. The problem was the elucidation of the part played by carbon in the long known corrosion of beryllium in CO_2-atmosphere. According to the overall equations:

$$Be + CO_2 \rightleftharpoons BeO + CO$$

and

$$Be + CO \rightleftharpoons BeO + C$$

carbon could be formed which might react further to give beryllium carbide. An answer was sought also to the question whether the carbon or the carbide on the beryllium surface is oxidised through carbon dioxide to carbon monoxide. Corroded sites should then contain accordingly more or less carbon which could be easily detected autoradiographically.

McCoy [301] maintained rotating beryllium samples, 1.25 cm diameter and 2.5 cm long, for longer periods in dry CO_2 at temperatures near to 1000° C. The CO_2 contained about 5% ^{14}C, prepared by thermal decomposition of Ba $^{14}CO_3$. After this corrosion treatment, the samples had to be polished for the subsequent work. The reaction with water of any Be_2C possibly formed ($Be_2C + 2H_2O \rightarrow 2BeO + CH_4$) during this polishing in a mixture of dry ethylene glycol and aluminium enery had to be avoided. It was found that the usual stripping film method used in metal autoradiography could not be employed on account of the reaction of beryllium with photographic developers. Only a method could be considered in which the photographic emulsion was separable from the preparation before development. McCoy used *Kodak-NTB*-film plates of 10 μ thickness of emulsion. Figs 10a and 10b show two highly magnified sections of the contact autoradiograms thus obtained. One can see clearly from the parallel dark patches of Figure (10a) that corrosion extends in one favoured direction. Figure 10b reproduces the autoradiogram of a surface at right angles to the plane of Figure 10a. The point-like cross-section of the sites of corrosion are recognisable. Corrosion manifestly begins at a narrowly circumscribed point. It extends longitudinally appreciably faster than transversely as a result of anisotropy of the material, probably determined by fault points. The corroded sites show up autoradiographically through their powerful contrast. A reaction, $Be + CO_2 \rightarrow BeO + CO$, predominant amongst those leading to corrosion, can thus be excluded; so much radiocarbon would not be present then. Whether the carbon in the corroded material is combined as Be_2C or occurs free cannot be decided from the autoradiogram alone when, as in the present example, work is carried out under exclusion of moisture.

Battery research is also availing itself increasingly of autoradiographic methods in order to investigate corrosion processes, regeneration processes in dry cells, sulphation of plates in the lead accumulator or electrochemical activity of gas electrodes [447; 127].

Herrmann and co-workers [191; 489; 187] followed the migration of antimony in the lead accumulator with the help of ^{124}Sb. Antimony has

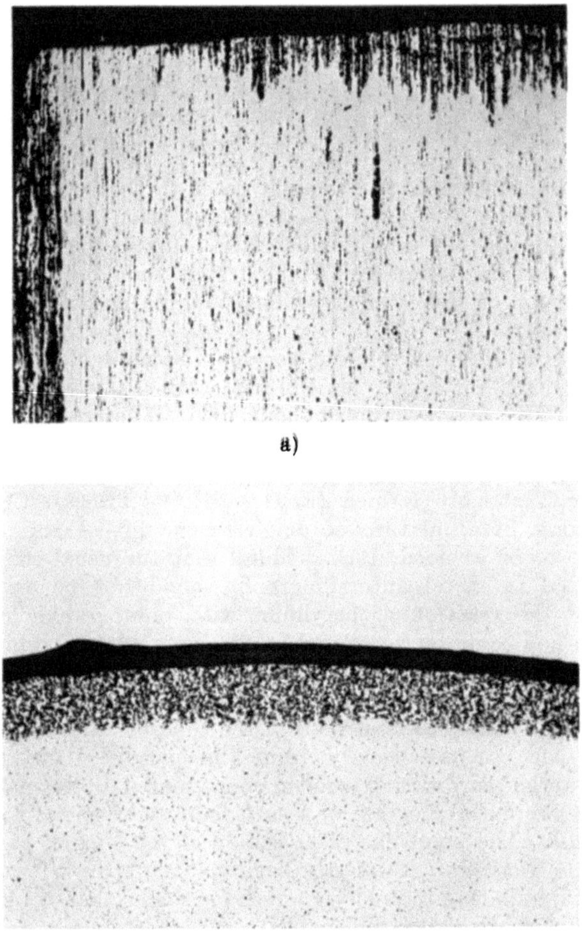

a)

b)

Fig. 10. Sections of the autoradiograms of a corroded beryllium sample, exposed for 355 hours to a $^{14}CO_2$ atmosphere at 704° C. From McCoy [301]
a) longitudinal; b) transverse direction of polishing

an unfavourable influence on the self-discharge of the plates and the gas emission at the negative plate is enhanced. Bode and Euler [59] studied local distribution of sulphate deposition. The plates were discharged in sulphuric acid which had been labelled with ^{35}S (Fig. 11). Selenium, the chemical compounds of which have properties similar to those of analogous sulphur compounds, was used also, as ^{75}Se. It is superior to ^{35}S since it is a soft γ-emitter and is thus autoradiographically detectable from a greater depth in the plates.

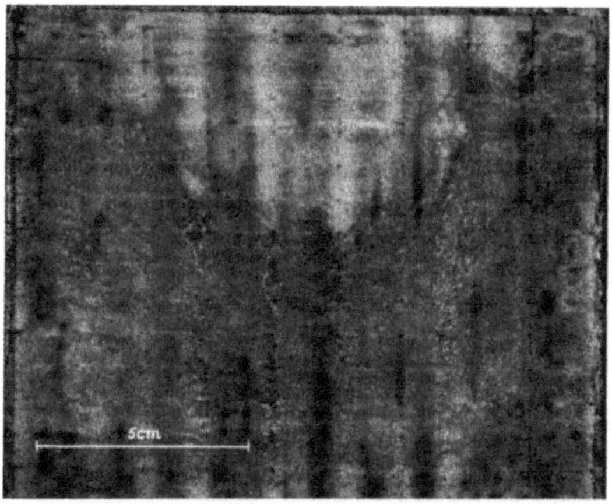

Fig. 11. Autoradiogram of a positive grid plate (section) from a lead accumulator. According to BODE and EULER [59]. Light patches correspond to deposition of $PbSO_4$ containing ^{35}Pb

4.1.5. Precipitates and inclusions in metals

Radioisotopes in autoradiographic techniques have proved valuable for detection and identification of inclusions in metals. The usual procedure, as described in the preceding examples, is to label radioactively each time one component of the material under investigation. It is more difficult when only a single metal sample is to be studied and a resmelt must not be performed. Neutron activation of the material often helps here (see Section 4.1.1.). MAKIN quotes a noteworthy variant, termed by him *extraction replica technique* [280]. Not the specimen itself is directly irradiated by neutrons but an etched surface replica. The etched, plane, specimen surface is given a thin film of formvar by spraying with a solution of formvar in chloroform. After the solvent has evaporated, the film is strengthened with a collodion layer from a solution in acetone. The parts of the double membrane which are of interest are separated with a razor blade. This furnishes a replica of the surface under investigation, with tiny dissolved traces of material through the preceding etching. This replica is irradiated with neutrons, regulated so that the carrier films do not become brittle. The irradiated replica is attached to a glass slide with acetone, covered with stripping film, exposed in the usual way and photographically developed. The replicas can be analysed γ-spectrometrically. Analyses of this sort are needed to eliminate interference with the results by impurities in the collodion or formvar. Inclusions of naturally radioactive substances can be analysed using the replica method, also without neutron activation. BIERLEIN and MASTEL [51] quote newer applications and also the adaption to smaller, light-microscopic specimens.

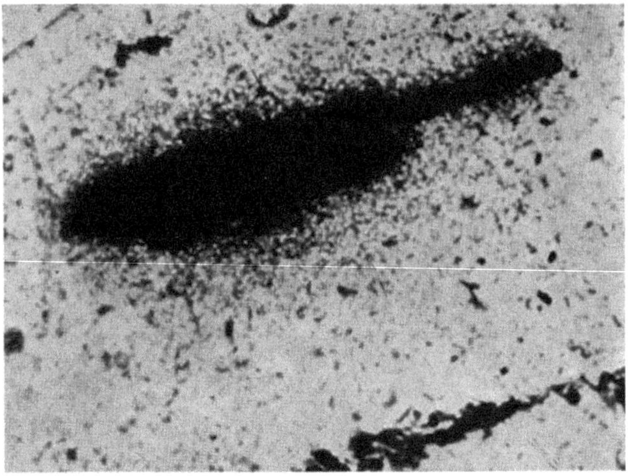

Fig. 12. Replica-autoradiogram of a manganese inclusion in steel, according to MAKIN [280]. The inclusion was identified through γ-spectrometric analysis as ^{56}Mn, derived from ^{55}Mn. Magnification: 400

4.2. Applications in chemical analysis

In practice, chemical and especially biochemical analysis involves detection of very small amounts of substances. These often occur together with other material from which they must first be separated, e. g., by chromatography or electrophoresis. The limit of detection is usually determined by the sensitivity of chemical tests, such as colour reactions. The limit can generally be reduced by radioactively labelling the substance and then detecting it autoradiographically. This type of method proved useful in the elucidation of the mechanism of photosynthesis, for instance; radioactive starting materials were used and very small amounts of intermediates in the synthesis could therefore be detected (Fig. 13).
Which autoradiographic method is best in any particular case is governed by the nature of the stationary phase employed in the chromatography or electrophoresis; this may be paper, thin-layer material, starch, cellulose or other gel-like substances.

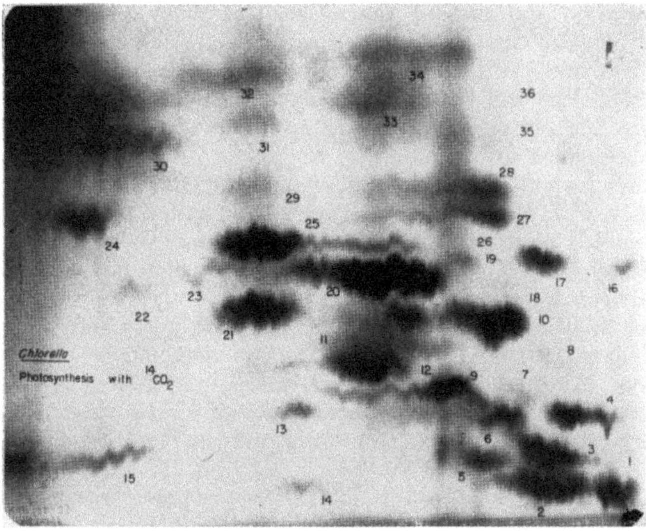

Fig. 13. Autoradiogram of a two-dimensionally developed paper chromatogram containing products of photosynthesis of *Chlorella* algae with $^{14}CO_2$. Film material: Kodak Single-Coated Blue-Sensitive Medical X-Ray Film; Time of Exposure: 8 days. From Moses et al [314]

4.2.1. Autoradiography of paper

The standard method for detecting labelled substances on dry chromatogram- or electrophoresis paper is to expose to it an X-ray film which is gently but steadily pressed against it. Very long exposure times are often needed for tritium-containing compounds since paper appreciably absorbs β-radiation of low energy. Further, the fibrous surface of the paper militates against good contact.

Wilson [482; 483] describes the preparation of autoradiograms in vessels with scintillator solutions. This reduces the time of exposure. The paper chromatogram is placed on a flat support and covered with a scintillator solution, e. g., 5 g 2,5-diphenyloxazole (*PPO*) or 3 g terphenyl in 1 litre toluene. So-called secondary scintillators, which adapt the primarily emitted light to the maximum sensitivity of the film, can be added also, e. g., 0.3 g/l of 4-methyl-5-phenyloxazolylbenzene (*dimethyl-POPOP*) or 0.01 g/l of diphenylhexatriene. The chromatograms should be marked so as to prevent confusion and also to fix the attachment of film and paper in each case. Radioactive strips of paper or foil or ink are suitable for this; the last named can be particularly useful in autoradiographic experiments [149; 202]. The most sensitive X-ray film possible, e. g., *Kodak Blue Band*, is then laid on the

chromatogram and pressed against it. One must ensure that all air bubbles between film and chromatogram are expelled. After exposure, the film is rinsed with water, cautiously freed from adhering solvent with a soft cloth and photographically developed.
Exposure in scintillator solutions is practicable only for detecting substances which are insoluble in the solvent used, toluene. In other procedures for autoradiography of paper-like materials, complete impregnation with photoemulsion is used. ROGERS [367] dipped the paper into a melted photographic emulsion and obtained quite good results with *nuclear research emulsion K2* (Ilford). This emulsion was developed especially for detection of low-energy radiation and has relatively little background. The emulsion was diluted 1:1 with water before immersion of the paper. 0.01 μC of a tritiated substance could be detected in a few days. Autoradiography seems rather pointless here, however; activities of this order can be measured and localised far faster nowadays by radio-paper chromatography, using windowless gas counting tubes.
A variant of ROGERS' procedure is spraying the paper with the emulsion instead of immersion in it. MARKMANN [289] uses Emulsion *G5* (Ilford), melting it at 50° C and diluting it 1:7 with water. 400 cm² of paper surface can be sprayed with 10 ml of this solution. Nitrogen or carbon dioxide are used as propellent gas. The emulsion is best dried in electrically heated vessels containing the drying agent calcium chloride. The dried papers are exposed in aluminium foil.

Table 3

Limits of detection of tritium on paper chromatograms. Values denoted with * have been estimated

Technique	Author(s)	Limit of detection μC/cm² and day
Contact exposure with X-ray film in liquid scintillator	WILSON [483]	0.2
Impregnation with liquid emulsion (Ilford *K2*)	ROGERS [367]	0.28
Impregnation with liquid emulsion (Ilford *G5*)	MARKMANN [289]	0.3
Contact exposure with *NTB* (Kodak)	SHEPPARD et al [408]	ca 0.3*
Contact exposure with X-ray film	RICHARDSON et al [364]	ca 0.4*
Contact exposure with X-ray film	CHAMBERLAIN et al [83]	0.28
Impregnation with Ilford *XK*	CHAMBERLAIN et al [83]	0.033

The emulsion *XK* (Ilford) has brought a decisive improvement in tritium detection on paper from chromatography and electrophoresis. CHAMBERLAIN, HUGHES, ROGERS and THOMAS [83] used it, based on the impregnation procedures of ROGERS [367] and MARKMANN [289]. It is interesting that CHAMBERLAIN et al also found X-ray films to be relatively sensitive towards tritium. Table 3 summarises the attainable sensitivities of detection, taken from various authors and based on various procedures.

^{32}P-[200] and ^{14}C-chromatograms demand no special devices for increasing sensitivity since their radiation energy is high. X-ray films are pressed firmly against the papers during exposure. The necessary exposure times can be gauged from the diagram given by GRENNEN TSUK et al [166] (Fig. 14).

Since paper is used to separate organic compounds mainly, labelling through neutron activation is practically restricted to phosphorus-containing substances. Neutron activation requires extremely clean paper, which is best purified again before irradiation. Soaking in formaldehyde and subsequently washing with water is suggested. According to JOHNSON, WEBER, CARTER and KROBER [218], phospho-

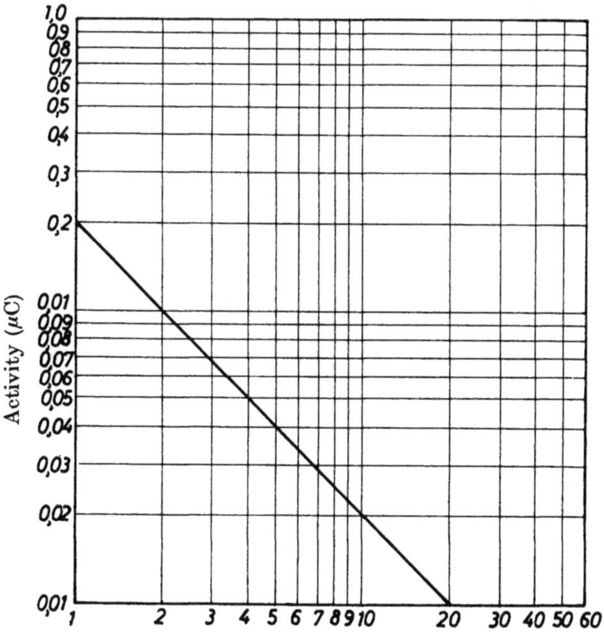

Fig. 14. Diagram for estimating the exposure time for paper chromatograms containing radiocarbon, according to GRENNEN TSUK et al [166]. Film material: X-ray film

lipoids, separated by paper chromatography, can be activated by IR-radiation with thermal neutrons (2.10^{12} n/m^2 sec.; 7 hours). A 48-hour interval between the end of irradiation and autoradiographic exposure is recommended in order to reduce background. Most of the short-life active radiation products decay during this period. Wooden frames (Fig. 15) which can be folded together have proved useful for the exposure; they facilitate good contact between paper and film [203].

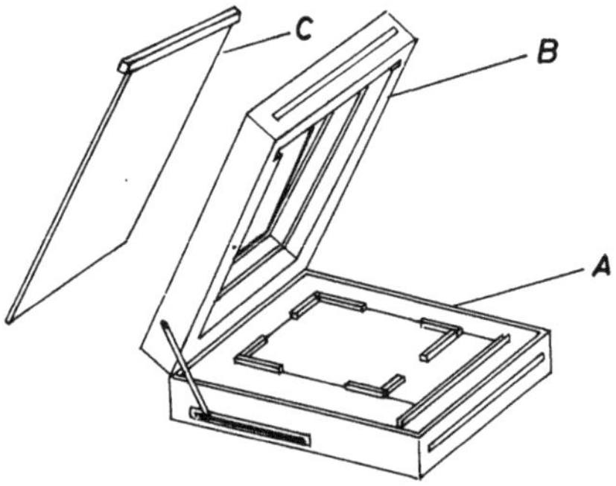

Fig. 15. Film holder for autoradiography of thin layer plates. The lower compartment A takes the plates (20 × 20 cm). The lid B contains the film cassette with a light-tight slide C for closing

Taken from E. Stahl: Thin layer Chromatography. Springer-Verlag, Berlin—Heidelberg—New York 1969, p. 158

4.2.2. Autoradiography of thin layers

The sharpness of resolution is less important than the sensitivity of detection in autoradiography of thin layers. The layers are claimed to absorb β-radiation rather less than does paper. The absorption of silica gel G and cellulose layers corresponds to a mass density of 5.5 and 7.5 mg/cm^2, respectively. This means, for instance, that over 95% of the tritium β-radiation is completely absorbed [212]. The layer easily suffers mechanical damage. This must be guarded against by appropriately careful handling. It is best to make use of special framing devices for holding plate and film. Several have been described, e. g., by Richardson, Weliky, Batchelder, Griffith and Engel [364]. The firm of G. Pleuger, Turnhoutsebaan, Belgium, sells a cassette suitable for holding thin layer plate and film (Fig. 15). According to Erismann [125], several plates and films may be exposed together autoradiographically as a multiple "sandwich."
The autoradiographical detection of tritium is harder than that of radiocarbon on thin layers just as on paper [287]. According to Chamberlain et al [83], direct immersion of the layer in photographic

emulsions cannot be considered since it is too easily damaged and also on account of chemographic effects. The sensitivity of detection of tritium can be increased by mixing silica gel G with anthracene. A 1:1 mixture (by weight) fluoresces in the presence of tritium. The light yield rises markedly as the temperature falls to —70° C [275]. Exposure is carried out at —40° C [276] (Fig. 16).

The "*Omnispray*" (Firm of New England Nuclear, Boston, USA) functions according to the same principle of radiation amplification. It has recently become available for contact autoradiography of tritium-containing substances on thin layers and paper. By spraying, the exposure time with silica gel layers is claimed to be reducible to a hundredth of that otherwise normally needed. Measurable autoradiographic blackening is then given by 0.1 μC ^{3}H in 16 hours [321]. For preparing the layers, the silica gel/anthracene mixture is ground in a ball mill to a grain size of 5 μ and less. 30 g of this powder are mixed into a sludge with 80 ml ethanol and applied to five 20 $\times$ 20 cm glass plates, yielding layers 0.25 mm thick. The layers are air dried. Solvents customarily used with silica gel G layers can be employed with this mixed layer. The separation efficiency is scarcely impaired.

Chemographic effects can be prevented by covering the layer with a sheet of plastic. Schwane and Nakon [403] give a procedure for this, applicable also to water-soluble compounds. In view of the long times of exposure, one ought to check whether it is not better to replace the thin layer autoradiography by the liquid scintillator technique.

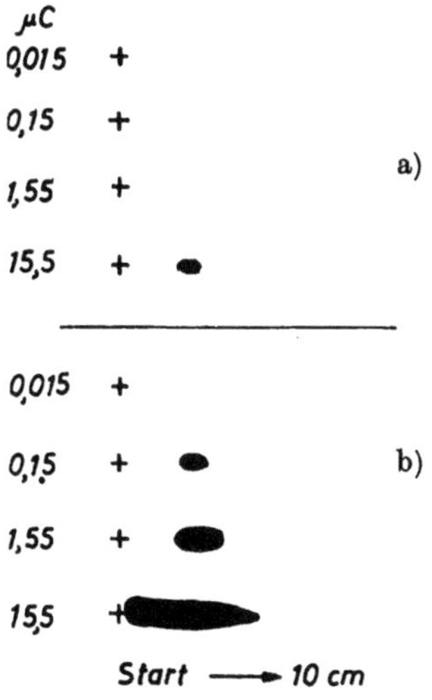

Fig. 16. Comparison between a normal thin-layer autoradiogram (a) and a fluoroautoradiogram (b) (Lüthi and Waser [275]). Substance: ^{3}H-diallylnortoxiferine. Film: *Kodirex* (Eastman Kodak)

Detection of ^{14}C-, ^{32}P-, ^{35}S-, ^{125}I- or ^{135}I-labelled substances is a wholly different matter; practically any film material is suitable for these [296]. Provided no chemographic effects occur through direct contact of the photographic film with the thin layer or with any substances in it, the air-dried layers can simply be covered with ordinary or X-ray film at room temperature. Another glass plate laid on top ensures sufficiently good and uniform contact. The commercially available, light-tight cassettes mentioned above facilitate storage during exposure in routine applications of autoradiography.

Fray and Frey [142] were able to shorten markedly the exposure time for thin layer chromatograms by varying the composition of the usual developer for X-ray film; this is tantamount to increasing the sensitivity of detection of ^{14}C-labelled substances (Table 4).

Table 4

Developer according to Fray and Frey [142]

Sodium sulphite (anhydrous)	100 g
Hydroquinone	4 g
Sodium borate	2.25 g
Boric acid	7 g
Phenidone (Geigy, Basel)	0.4 g

The compounds in Table 4 are dissolved in that order in water at 45° C and the solution made up to 1 litre with distilled water. The development time for *Isopan Record* (Agfa) (1250 ASA = 32° DIN), for example, is 12—13 min at 20°. This developer is claimed to increase the sensitivity by a factor of 8 to 32, compared with the standard developer *D 19* (Kodak). This increased sensitivity is of course at the expense of some loss in contrast and gradation of the image, in other words, diminished resolution. This is not so tragic with thin layer chromatograms, however, since interest is centred only on detection and approximate

Table 5

Sensitivity of detection of ^{14}C-containing substance spots on thin layer chromatograms

Time of contact (hours)	Detectable ^{14}C amount	
	μC	$\mu C/cm^2$
0.5	0.5	0.21
1	0.01	0.05
2	0.005	0.04
6	0.0025	0.016
24	0.0005	0.0026
268	0.00005	0.0003

localisation of active material; spots with a cross section smaller than 1 mm are not found in any case.
Table 5 gives the dependence of the lower limit of ^{14}C detection on the time of exposure, taken from FRAY and FREY's thin layer autoradiograms. The values are for cellulose layers. It can be seen that 0.3 nC of $^{14}C/cm^2$ can still be detected after about 11 days exposure (Fig. 17).

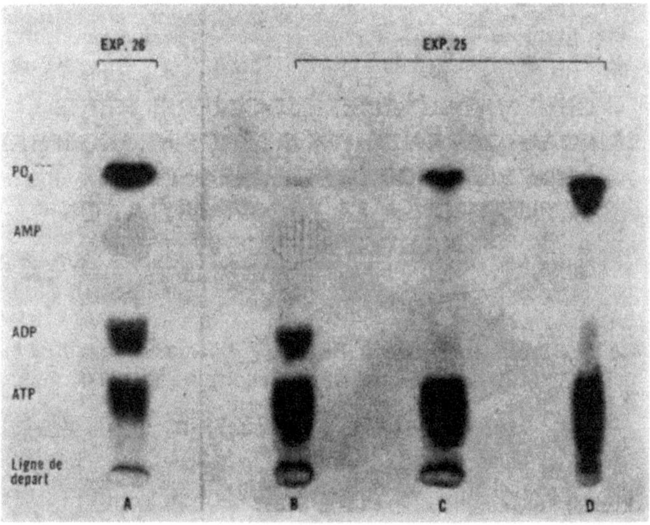

Fig. 17. Autoradiogram of a cellulose thin-layer, prepared for determination of some adenosine phosphates formed by photophosphorylation from $H_3{}^{32}PO_4$ in the presence of myokinase. From BOVE [64]

Differentiation is sometimes possible where different isotopes have been used for labelling. For example, a chromatogram containing ^{14}C- and ^{32}P-compounds can be exposed to X-ray film immediately and again after several months. The blackening of the first autoradiogram is due to the radiation from both isotopes; that of the second, only to radiocarbon, since the other isotope has sensibly entirely decayed.
Another method for detecting two emitters present together is based on the differing radiation energies. Two X-ray films are placed one above the other on a chromatogram containing, e. g., ^{14}C- and ^{32}P-labelled substances. After development, the film nearer to the chromatogram shows the positions of spots containing both isotopes; that further away, only the spots containing ^{32}P because the radiation from ^{14}C has a shorter range and does not pass right through the first film.
Yet another possibility is to screen the soft radiation of radioactive sulphur and carbon from that of phosphorus by means of a thin (0.1 mm) aluminium sheet. ^{131}I can also be detected in presence of ^{35}P or ^{14}C in

this way. RICHARDSON, WELIKY, BATCHELDER, GRIFFITH and ELDER [364] describe screening the softer radiation of ^3H by cellophane in order to separate it from that of ^{14}C. BUCKALOV and COHN [68] worked with colour films in *colour autoradiography* for multiple labelling. This depends on radiations of different energies from the various isotopes yielding recognisably different colours.

So far, neutron activation does not appear to have been applied in the realm of thin layer chromatography. Many elements are present in adsorbent, binder and glass and this leads to formation of a large number of isotopes of various lengths of life. This impedes autoradiographic detection of spots of substances present only in traces.

The work of LAMBIOTTE [248; 249; 250] is worth mentioning on account of its originality. He tested the possibilities of thin layer electrophoresis-autoradiography in a photographic film, saturated with a buffer solution. The autoradiogram functioned as stationary phase. He used *Kodirex X-ray Film* (Kodak). After electrophoretic separation of the radioactive substance, the film was exposed for several days. A relatively high sensitivity of detection results from the internal contact between the radiation-sensitive substance and the radiation-sensitive material: 10^{-3} μC of a tritiated compound can be detected after 6 days exposure. The procedure is recommended in particular for determining radioactive impurities in radiochemicals (Figs 18 & 19).

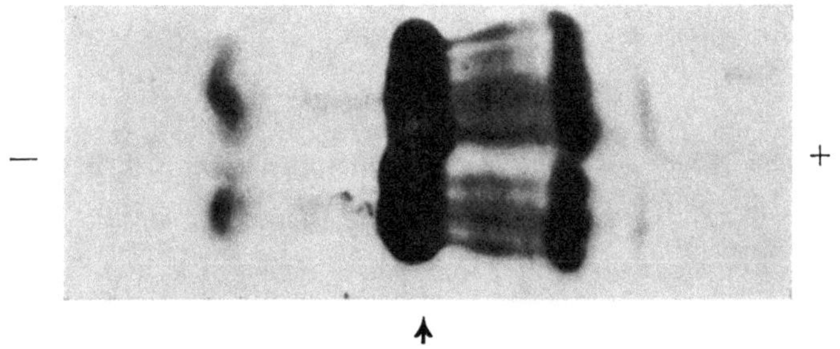

Fig. 18. Impurities in ^3H-methionine, resulting from autoradiolysis. Detection through thin layer electrophoresis-autoradiography according to LAMBIOTTE [250]

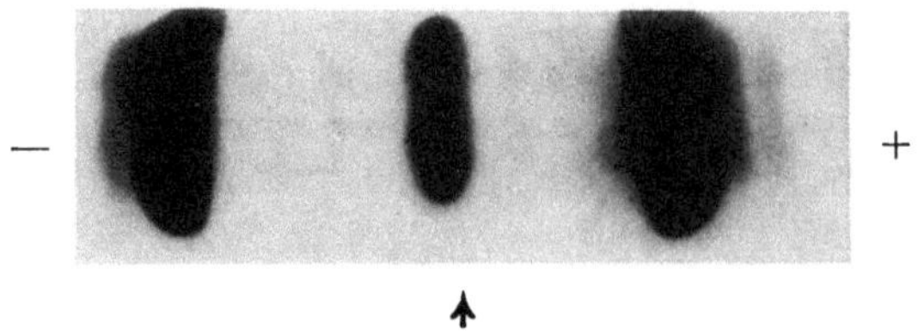

Fig. 19. Separation of ^{14}C-histidine, ^3H-valine and ^{14}C-glutamic acid by electrophoresis-autoradiography according to LAMBIOTTE [250]. Arrows indicate the position of spotting

4.2.3. Biochemical analysis and immunology

Numerous investigations have been carried out on blood serum using autoradiography, mostly following electrophoresis [31]. The fractions thus separated are often characterised through their affinity to iodide or Fe^{2+} ions. The use of radioactive nuclides, such as ^{125}I, ^{131}I or ^{59}Fe, facilitates detection of the corresponding fractions when appropriate radiation measuring apparatus is employed; and also increases sensitivity of detection, in conjunction with autoradiography. Further, this principle may provide quantitative information about capacities for bond and metabolic activities [186].

Dessauer, Fox and Hartwig [99] detected autoradiographically the transferrins (a term for all serum proteins which combine with iron) of 150 different species of reptile and amphibian in relation to their taxonomy and ecological factors. Investigations of this sort can be significant for estimating the degree of relationship of individual species. For preparing the autoradiograms, 2 μl plasma are mixed with 0.2 to 1 μC (10 to 50 μl) of a 0.012 mM ferrous sulphate solution containing $^{59}Fe^{2+}$. This solution is submitted to electrophoresis for 17—20 hours on starch gel layers. The gel layer is then cut across with a steel wire of 0.2 mm diameter. One half of the layer is stained in the usual way with the protein-specific dye amido black; the other half is wrapped in a plastic film (*Saran-polyethylene* of the Dow Chemical Corporation). This plastic covering prevents the layer from drying out and at the same time protects it from undesirable chemographic effects during the subsequent exposure for 1—2 days at +10° C. Commercial X-ray film holders can be used for this (*X-ray Exposure Holder*, Eastman-Kodak).

Roy and Neuhaus [388] modified the procedure by using acetic acid-methanol-water (1+5+5) to fix previously the half of the layer destined for autoradiography. When the autoradiogram is compared with the electropherogram, the shrinkage of the starch layer during staining must be allowed for (Fig. 20).

The operational technique is complicated by division of the starch gel layer into two parts which are subsequently treated differently. Jackson [213] describes a less tedious method in which the dried starch gel layer ($\frac{3}{16}$ inch thick) is autoradiographed directly. After electrophoretic separation of the serum containing $^{59}FeSO_4$, the gel layer is covered with a film of plastic. Gas bubbles and irregularities are removed by careful rubbing. The rest of the "sandwich" consists of X-ray film, glass plate and a lead weight (Fig. 21).

The passage of radiation between preparation and photographic layer is weakened only negligibly by the plastic foil. ^{59}Fe is a relatively strong γ-emitter ($E\gamma = 1.1$ and 1.29 MeV) and also a β-emitter ($E_{max} = 0.46$ and 0.27 MeV). Autoradiographic resolution is governed in this case entirely by the γ-components of the radiation and is scarcely affected by the inserted foil. The electropherogram is stained with amido black

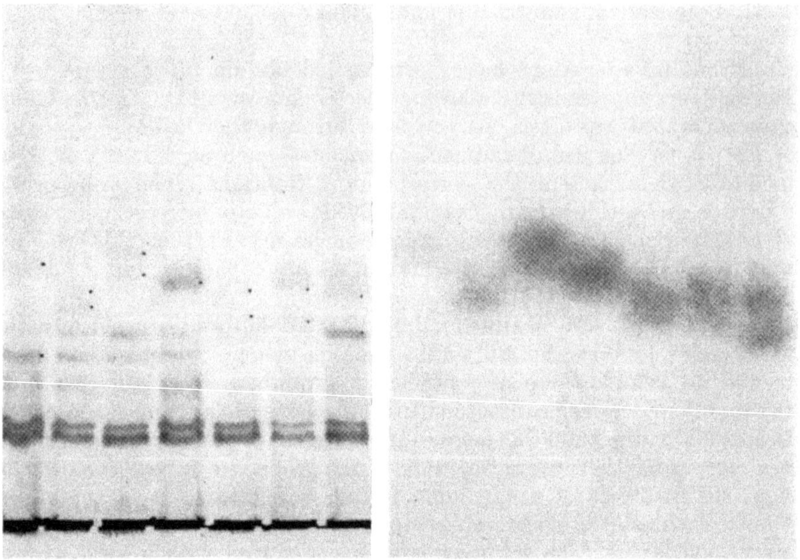

Fig. 20. Intraspecific transferrin variants in *Coluber constrictor*
Left: stained starch gel electropherogram of plasma samples from 7 species of animal;
Right: autoradiogram of the zones containing ^{59}Fe.
The points in the left-hand figure denote the site of transferrins detected autoradiographically. From [99]

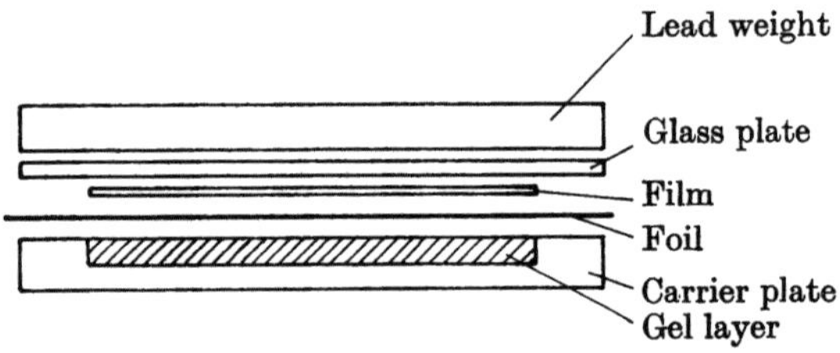

Fig. 21. Exposure of starch gel layers for autoradiography after Jackson [213]

in the usual way after autoradiographic exposure. If staining is done beforehand, exposure times are about doubled, presumably due to soluble radioactive material having been washed out.

Autoradiography finds analytical application in *immunology* also. Usually it is a question of detection or identification of zones in which protein fractions coincide in electrophoresis [42] or through diffusion [338] and react or agglutinate to soluble or insoluble complexes. The fractions are generally tagged with a radioactive iodine isotope [186; 380], the presence of which does not significantly modify the chemical and physical properties of the protein macromolecule. Agar gel serves as carrier for these processes. In the dry state it may be brought into direct contact with the film without danger of chemography [348]. The best autoradiographic results have been obtained with X-ray films because energy-richer emitters, such as iron or iodine isotopes, can be used in biochemical investigations with natural products.

4.3. Application to biological specimens

4.3.1. General comments

In principle, any autoradiographic technique can be applied to study biological specimens. At the moment, however, there is a growing tendency to replace the use of liquid photographic emulsions (i. e., the "*coated* procedure" of BÉLANGER and LEBLOND [40]) and of simple photographic plates (e. g. in the contact or "*mounted* procedure" of EVANS [128]) by the *stripping film* technique of PELC [343]. An exception is the autoradiography of water-soluble substances, for which the stripping film technique is unsuitable (moist film material has to be laid on the specimen). One can use only contact procedures here. Such methods have proved satisfactory also for those biological specimens where the excessive size of the preparation surface renders application of stripping film impracticable. Liquid emulsions can perhaps still be employed with specimens having an uneven surface (cf Section 4.5.).
The autoradiography of larger biological specimens serves primarily for acquiring a rough, preliminary idea and picture of the distribution in the organism of each applied radioactive substance and its metabolites; short exposure times are thus of interest. Relatively coarse-grained, sensitive plates of X-ray films are used, which, because of this, have low resolution.
The resolution of the "classical" contact method, i. e., autoradiography by laying a photographic plate on the even-surfaced preparation under investigation, is, for β-emitters such as tritium or radiocarbon, about 20 to 100 μ, depending on experimental conditions. The blackening on the autoradiogram within a radius of this size permits the position of the source of radiation in the preparation to be determined. This resolution limit satisfies the requirements of studies on larger specimens, as stated above (Section 4.2.). If the preparations are especially thin and have extremely smooth surfaces and there is good contact between them and the films, the contact procedure allows allocations extending into the cell region (cf Section 5.4.3.).
For mechanical and technical reasons, the thickness of the preparation cannot be reduced indefinitely. Further, it is found in practice that

increase in the surface area of the section inevitably has an influence on the thickness. Using ultramicrotomes and specimens embedded in plastic, sections of a few hundred Å thickness can be prepared. Larger-surfaced specimens, however, can at best be cut in sections a few μ thick. This thickness is, however, enough to satisfy the needs for autoradiography of such specimens.
Biological specimens on which autoradiographic studies are pursued can be classified as follows, according to their nature and size:

1. Organ and tissue samples,
2. Preparations of various mechanical consistencies,
3. Bones and cartilage,
4. Animals (e. g., mice, rats).

Apart from the first group, which is discussed in Chapter 5, the preparations (i. e., of groups 2, 3 and 4) are, without exception, larger specimens. In the following pages are discussed problems which arise in connection with their preparation for autoradiographic investigation; and also ways and possibilities of solving these problems. A detailed description of histological techniques cannot, however, be undertaken*.

4.3.2. Preparation of larger specimens for autoradiographic investigation

In the preparation of biological samples for autoradiographic study, it is vitally important to suppress as far as humanly possible any displacement of the labelled substances to be detected, after the sample has been taken from the animal or it has been killed. This is possible practically only through the freeze technique and is particularly advisable when the tagged substance is not structurally bound and occurs originally in the cell in soluble, so-called diffusible, form (cf Section 5.4.). Diffusion is largely retarded by rapid freezing of the tissue ("freeze shock"), as a rule without tissue and cell structure suffering changes that are detectable light-microscopically. Freezing can be carried out in two ways, both giving satisfactory results:

1. Small specimens, e. g., individual organs, can be relatively simply and rapidly frozen with carbon dioxide delivered from a steel cylinder; as a result of the sudden fall in pressure, some solid carbon dioxide "snow" is yielded. The specimen to be frozen is laid on a "freeze block" and frozen to moistened paper which has previously been placed on

---

* Histological techniques are treated for example in: H. Adam und G. Czihak: Arbeitsmethoden der makroskopischen und mikroskopischen Anatomie. G. Fischer Verlag, Stuttgart 1964. Romeis, B.: Mikroskopische Technik. R. Oldenbourg Verlag, München-Wien 1968. Burck, H.-C.: Histologische Technik. G. Thieme Verlag, Stuttgart 1966.

the block. The frozen material can be easily handled together with the block and fixed to the microtome. It is essential to wait until the temperature of the specimen has attained that within the cryostat before beginning sectioning. The frozen objects are best kept for several hours in firmly closed plastic bags, sealed hermetically as far as possible [481]. This packing largely prevents drying out. Some authors recommend covering the specimens with vaseline or coating their surface with paraffin-hexane (3+1) so that a paraffin film remains after the hexane has evaporated [437]. If such measures are not adopted, the surface of the specimen shrinks.

2. The alternative method of rapid freezing is to introduce the biological material into liquid air or into a hydrocarbon, e. g., isopentane, cooled in liquid air. Large specimens can, however, undergo macroscopic rupture of tissue through this sudden fall in temperature [437]. Acetone-dry ice mixtures and *Peltier* cascades [401] have been used also to freeze biological material.

The problem of cutting frozen biological material has been solved technically in a satisfactory way and presents no particular difficulties. Series of sections can be prepared in the laboratory in a reasonable time. Nowadays, several firms provide cryostats with built-in microtome. In most cases, the hands and forearms of the experimentor are

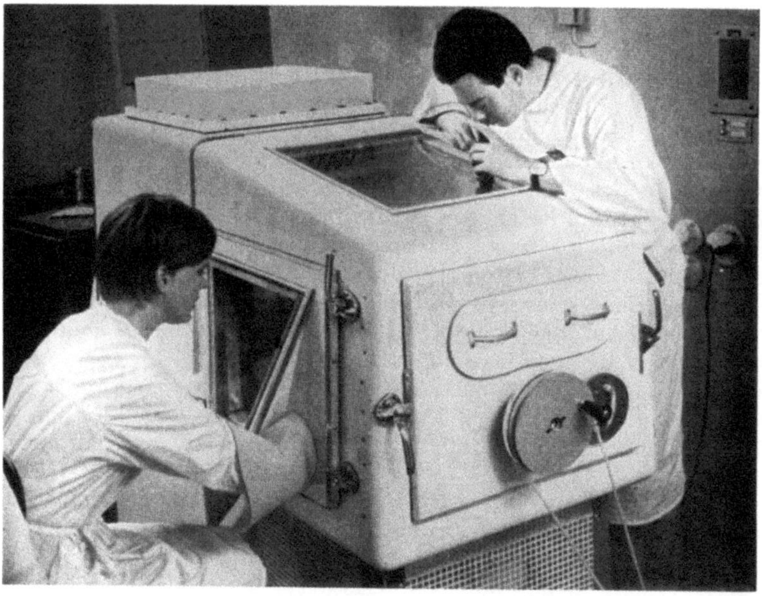

Fig. 22. Universal cryostat of the firm W. Dittes, Heidelberg, Germany, equipped with the minotmicrotome of the firm Jung of Heidelberg and with a microscope. The microtome is operated with a pedal. From [438]

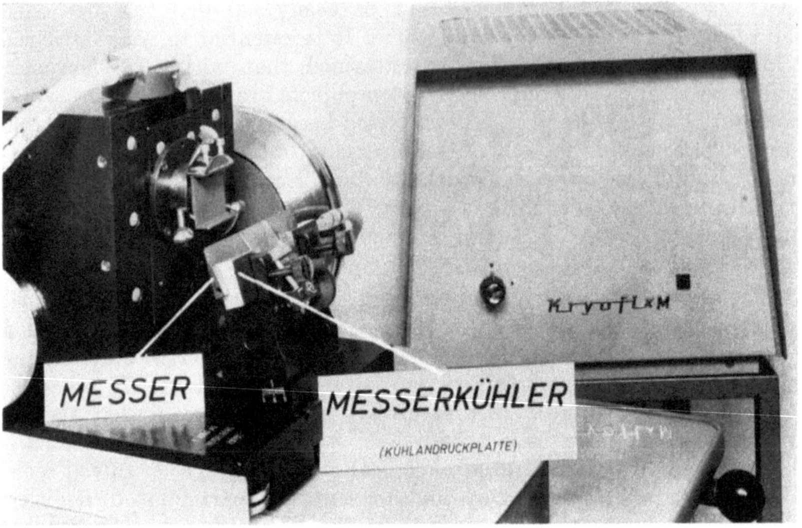

(Messer = knife, Messerkühler = knife-cooler)

Fig. 23. Inner view of the apparatus of Fig. 24. The cryotome with knife cooling and freezing block are recognisable

in a cool chamber fitted with a microtome for serial cutting, using external electric power. Large window openings enable all working operations to be observed (Fig. 22, 23, 24).

It is known that the melting point of water is lowered by increase in pressure. This explains why frozen biological material can be comparatively easily cut with a microtome. The tissue briefly thaws in the vicinity of the knife edge as a result of the pressure on it. Despite the relatively small force which the microtome knife exerts, the knife edge has a small area and the pressure produced is thus enormous. As soon as the knife has separated parts of the tissue and exerts no further pressure on them, they refreeze. Additional knife coolers are available in order to keep the zone as small as possible in which these transitions from solid to liquid state and back occur. These give the knife a lower temperature than the tissue. The sections then pass smoothly over the knife and this is claimed especially to facilitate cutting specimens of high fat content (Fig. 24).

Series of 3 to 8 μ thick sections can be taken without difficulty from specimens with a cross-section up to ca 5 cm^2. In contrast, however, suitable frozen sections cannot be obtained from larger specimens showing local variations in hardness and elasticity, without special aids. Increasing section thickness is no solution; this usually leads to its splitting. An effective trick which has often proved highly successful is to cover the surface of the specimen with thin adhesive tape, best

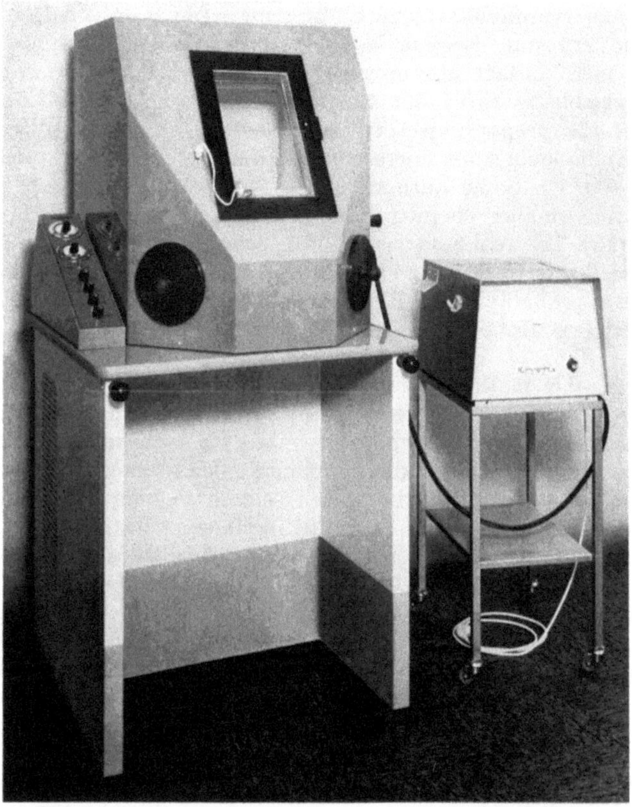

Fig. 24. WK-cryotome with knife cooler as auxiliary apparatus (firm WKF Brandau). The specimens can be frozen at temperatures down to —45° C in the apparatus, without using carbon dioxide. The cooling principle ensures constant and reproducible regulation of the section thickness from 40 μ down to about 1 μ

transparent. This prevents the separated section from disintegration and enables it to be more easily handled [449]. But even here transverse cracks may occur in the section. Some authors [438] circumvent the use of the relatively rigid adhesive film by employing a 50% solution of ethyl methacrylate in ethyl acetate. This is applied with a brush to the surface of the section (ca 0.02 ml/cm²). After about 15 min, during which the solvent evaporates, a thin, non-sticky coating remains adhering very firmly to the tissue. Section and film are raised during the passage of the microtome knife and retained on a suitably sized glass slide.

Frozen sections should be largely dried by storage in a cryostat before they are introduced into a normal air-conditioned space. Any condensation of atmospheric moisture on the specimen can be prevented by warming the slide and preparation to bring them up to room temperature with an electric microheater or by pressing a finger on it before removal from the cryostat. Section and photographic emulsion are usually brought into contact at ambient temperature. Yet, for two reasons, it is advisable to carry out this subsequent exposure at lower temperature: the preparation then keeps better, and the background of photographic emulsions increases less rapidly at lower temperature (+2 to +4° C). Some authors prefer temperatures down to —20° C, anticipating smaller chemographic effects as well as the lower background [13]. The real reason why it appears more sensible to maintain freeze-dried preparations at lower temperatures during autoradiographic exposure is probably because the preparation is thereby more effectively conserved (see also Section 5.4. 3.4.) and artefacts by crystals are not possible.

There are other methods for preparing thin sections of larger specimens than by employing the frozen section technique. Their suitability for autoradiographic purposes must be tested for each particular case. For example, it is possible to submit juvenile mice to vacuum freeze-drying and then to avoid using the frozen section technique by subsequent embedding in paraffin wax [449]. Cutting larger paraffin wax-embedded specimens is subject, however, to the same difficulties as those mentioned in connection with the frozen section principle; embedding in paraffin wax thus brings no particular advantages for histological preparation.

We cannot deal in more detail with the embedding procedures using organic polymers, frequently used in recent times. Each experimentor has his own "personal" mixture anyhow. The mechanical stability of the sections attained through embedding in plastic is undoubtedly superior to that from the frozen section technique. This gain is countered, however, by appreciably longer autoradiographic exposure times incurred through the increased absorption of radiation by the embedding medium-especially with tritium-containing material.

4.3.3. Preparations composed of hard and soft structures

Embedding in plastic has proved suitable for specimens, the structures of which are not uniformly hard and of the same mechanical consistency. Examples are the sinus regions with jawbones, teeth and gums. Sognnaes et al [420; 421] developed a special method for embedding and cutting preparations of this kind with subsequent autoradiography in mind. These authors used the liquid monomer, methyl methacrylate, which is polymerised by addition of the catalyst benzoyl peroxide after it has sufficiently penetrated and diffused into the tissue. Other descriptions of simple equipment and methods for embedding and preparing sections from brittle and fragile material are given by: Axelrod [19]; Laude, Janes and Boyd [253]; Myers, Jennings and Becks [315]; Woodruff and Norris [487]; and Norris and Jenkins [324]. An important prerequisite for autoradiographic investigations of dental metabolism has been realised through the development of such techniques [41; 36; 37; 228; 241; 199; 227; 465].

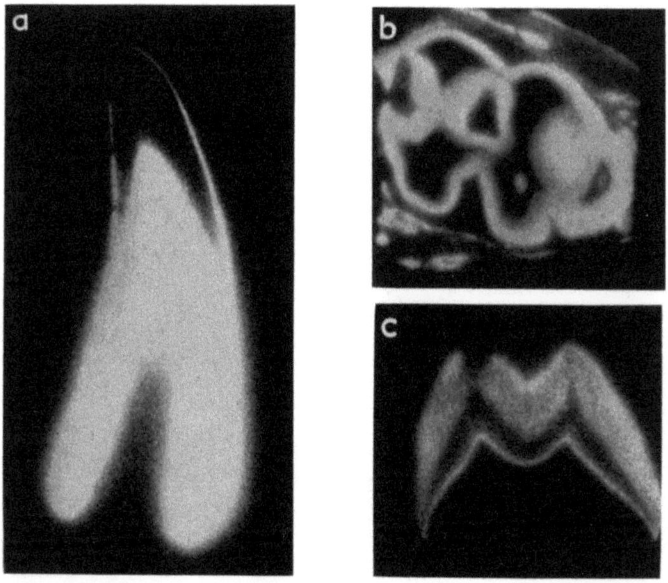

Fig. 25. Contact autoradiograms of plastic-embedded sections through jaw regions of Rhesus monkeys after injection of 15 mC of a ^{32}P-compound. From SOGNNAES et al [421]

a) Longitudinal section through a *Caninus*, not yet fully emerged, two days after injection. Extremely high concentration of ^{32}P at the tip of the root, in the predentine zone and in the surface of the enamel
b) Jaw section in the region of the not yet fully emerged third *molar*, nine days after injection. The activity of the calcifying enamel and of the bone is appreciably higher than that of the dentine
c) Longitudinal section through the region portrayed in b)

4.3.4. Bone and cartilage sections

Many chemical elements have a high affinity for bone tissue, i. e., they are taken up preferentially by bone. One refers to "bone-seeking" elements (Figs 26 & 27). This gains significance when one thinks of the uptake of radioactive elements and the action of their radiation on the organism, especially on the blood-forming centres*. Autoradiography

* A monograph on "Radiation, Isotopes and Bone" by F. C. McLEAN and A. M. BUDY, was published by Academic Press, N. Y. in 1964.

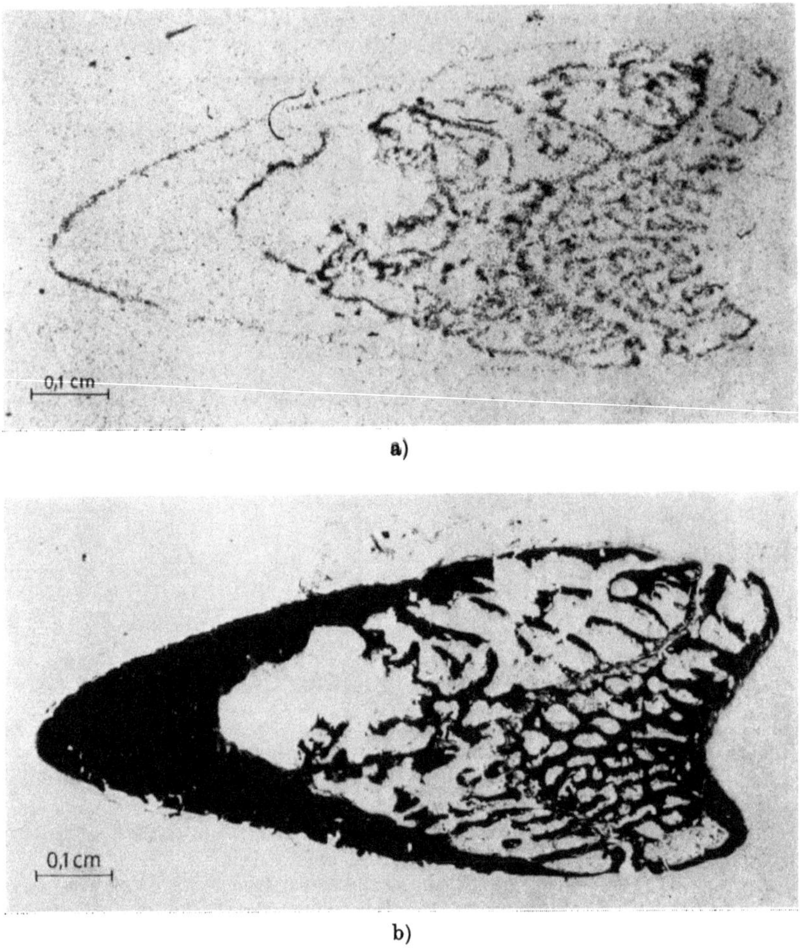

Fig. 26. Contact autoradiogram of the *femur* of an adult rat after injection of a few micrograms plutonium which belongs to the "bone-seeking" elements. Killed 8 days later. Note the accumulation on the surface of the shaft and trabecula and absence from the epiphyseal cartilage (a). The associated section (b) was stained with $AgNO_3$-haemotoxylin-eosin. From HAMILTON [177]

has played an important part in clearing up many problems [291; 292; 293; 294; 386; 387].

The quality and information value of bone autoradiograms depend decisively on correct preparation of the bone sections [67]. The bones under investigation should not be decalcified, even when no changes are to be feared in the structures in which interest is centred. There is

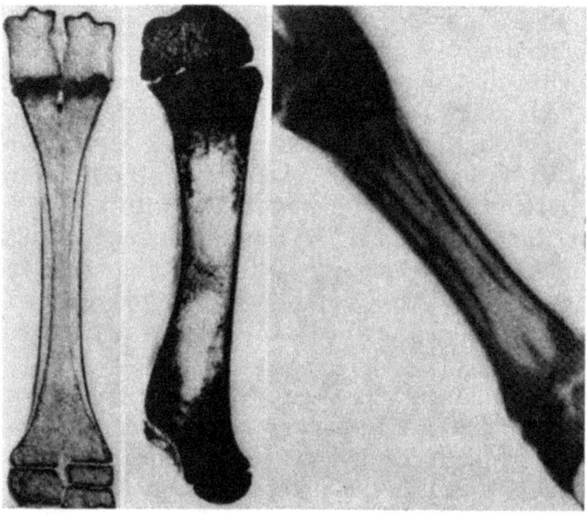

Fig. 27. Contact autoradiograms of bone sections according to LOTZ, GALLIMORE and BOYD [274]

a) *Metatarsus* of a calf after oral administration of 0.5 mC ^{45}Ca-compound that is not precisely designated. Exposure time of 15 days;
b) *Femur* of an 80-day old pig after intravenous administration of 0.25 mC ^{45}Ca-compound. Killed 10 days later. Exposure time of 13 days;
c) *Metatarsus* of a bull, 4.85 mC ^{90}Sr- and ^{90}Y-salt. Exposure time of 2 days

too grave a risk of dissolving radioactive substances during decalcification and thus of altering the distribution of activity in the preparation. LOTZ, GALLIMORE and BOYD [274] developed a device for preparing comparatively thin sections for autoradiographic studies on larger bones. A thickness of about 2 mm can be attained. Before cutting, the freshly prepared bones are cemented on to a smooth board with *Duco cement*; the long axis of the bone should be placed along the length of the board if possible. The cement sets overnight. It is better to use plaster of Paris with short-life isotopes or if displacements of the radioactive substances are feared, because it sets much faster. One can then begin cutting the bone only 30 minutes after applying the plaster of Paris. The authors used an electrically driven band saw for sectioning, sensibly devoid of vibration, for this purpose. The board, which is rigidly attached to the material to be cut and which must have an even external surface, permits the bone preparation to be easily handled during cutting. The board is moved along a guide rail, fixed firmly to the saw bench, so that an evenly cut surface results. Sections of various thicknesses can be prepared by displacing the rails parallel to the saw. The whole system is in a glove box, connected with an ordinary vacuum cleaner in order to avoid radioactive contamination through

sawdust and as a precaution against radiation. If a more precise histological evaluation of the bone section is desired, the specimen is best frozen with dry ice after the binder has set. Any sawdust contaminating the surface is carefully removed with a soft brush. Autoradiographic exposure is carried out with X-ray film in a light-tight cassette at —15 to —20° C; chemographic effects are avoided if necessary by separating film and preparation with thin plastic foil.
Earlier, Libby [268] had used a "section" technique, similar to that of Lotz et al, for preliminary cutting of deep-frozen whole animals. Relatively thick sections (ca 3—4 mm) were subsequently freeze dried, embedded in paraffin and reduced to about 1 mm thickness with a microtome.
Kalberer [222] used a circular saw for cutting animals which had been frozen in liquid air. The frozen body was then immersed in paper pulp. The paper coating which froze on to the specimen enabled it to be more easily handled. Above all, it was less susceptible to mechanical damage when fixed in a special holder on the saw bench (Fig. 28).

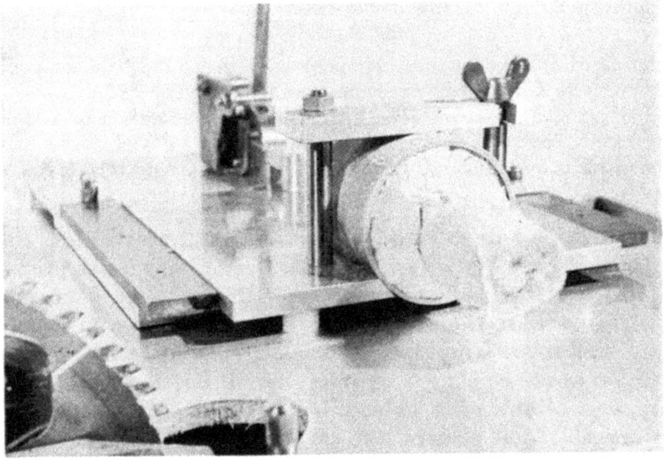

Fig. 28. Holder for deep-frozen specimens in preparation of whole body sections according to Kalberer [222]. The diagram shows an experimental animal cut transversely

The contact method in bone autoradiography has the great advantage of being simple and a suitable routine procedure. Preparation and autoradiogram can be separated after exposure and each handled further without mutual interference. The shortcoming of the method is the inferior resolution, due to the relatively poor contact between preparation and photographic layer. Cellular localisation of radioelements is not possible.

Hsieh, Hungate and Wilson [208] developed a technique especially for detecting α-emitters in bones. It enables the exposure time to be drastically reduced. They based their method on the fact that less than 100 eV are necessary to expose a silver halide grain (see Section 6.2.2.), i. e., more than 99% of the energy of an emitter of 5 MeV is ineffective. Accordingly, they attempted to raise the grain yield by an intermediate phosphor. As a suitable energy transformer, they found microcrystalline zinc sulphide containing traces of silver (ZnS: Ag P7—920B of the U. S. Radium Co.). 25 g of this sulphide were suspended in 100 ml of 2% aqueous gelatine solution and deposited directly on the bone section or on to a film sandwiched between specimen and photo-emulsion. This was an aluminium-coated *Mylar film* (1 mg/cm^2, of the Alexander Vacuum Co., USA) or of painted-on plastic. Polaroid photographic film was used instead of the otherwise usual Kodak film *NTA* or *NTB*. It was pressed gently against the preparation, as customary in contact autoradiography (Fig. 29). The exposure time required was about 1000 times smaller than with the films mentioned. The autoradiograms are thus ready in a few minutes, yet resolution is claimed to be only slightly inferior to that of the ordinary method. Apparatus is suggested for routine investigations in which the aluminium-plastic film with its zinc sulphide layer is placed directly opposite the open window of a polaroid film cassette. The sections studied need only to be pressed on to it (Fig. 29b). They can be exchanged rapidly at any

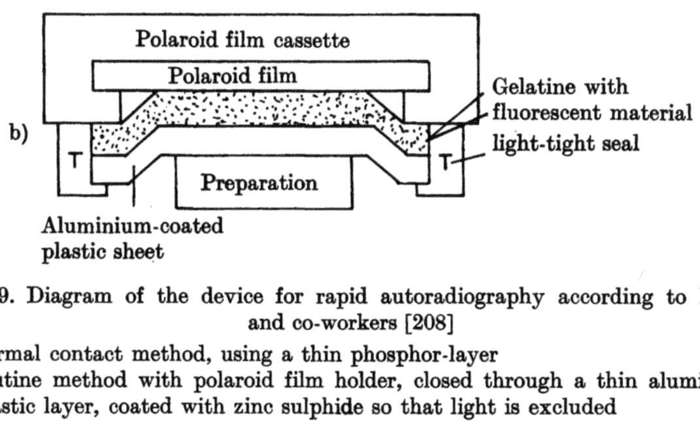

Fig. 29. Diagram of the device for rapid autoradiography according to Hsieh and co-workers [208]

a) normal contact method, using a thin phosphor-layer

b) routine method with polaroid film holder, closed through a thin aluminium-plastic layer, coated with zinc sulphide so that light is excluded

time in normal illumination and the autoradiogram is practically immediately available. *Polascope 410* or *Land 57*, both *positive* and *negative*, are used as film material.

We can quote only a few examples of the importance of autoradiography in research on structure and metabolism of bones and teeth. ERBACHER and WANNEMACHER [123] were the first to show that metabolic processes occur in enamel. COUCEIRO [86] demonstrated that dental metabolism occurs relatively rapidly. BARTELSTONE et al [29] discovered that a dynamic equilibrium exists between blood and teeth. More recently, autoradiography has been applied to study the calcium- and fluorine metabolism in teeth [28; 35; 465].

4.3.5. Whole-body autoradiography

The development of cutting technique and commercial availability of microtomes for serial cutting (Figs. 22, 24) have greatly furthered the autoradiography of larger biological specimens, notably of whole laboratory animals (whole-body autoradiography) [67]. An experimental animal is sectioned in a longitudinal or sagittal direction. The preparations thus yielded are heterogeneous and of low mechanical resistance, due to the many tissues and organs which they contain. They must be handled with great care, particularly in connection with autoradiographic operations. Since whole-body autoradiography is being used more and more in pharmacological research, it will be treated in detail in the following pages. We shall limit ourselves to the technique practised by ULLBERG. Almost all pertinent publications are of work based on this method. Mice, rats and guinea pigs are the animals most often used. In principle, still larger animals would be suitable also but the technical demands, difficulties and possibilities of error increase with increasing size of animal.

A microtome with a heavy sledge is required, e. g., of the type "Grundschlitten" (Firm of Leitz, Wetzlar, Germany), "K" or "Minot" (Firm of Jung, Heidelberg, Germany), which is built into a thermostated freezing cabinet (Fig. 22). The usual section thickness in whole-body autoradiography is ca 20 μ.

The experimental animal is frozen in either dry ice-hexane (—75° C) or isopentane-liquid nitrogen (—150° C). The animal body is frozen to the microtome block with the help of a viscous mixture of carboxymethylcellulose-water. Any surface thawing must be avoided. The temperature of the cryostat chamber should be at least —10° C. The preparation must be in thermal equilibrium with the cryostat and means must be found to prevent superficial drying out of the preparation before this equilibrium is established (see Section 4.3.2.).

It is advisable to use a miniature circular saw to prepare larger animals for sectioning (Fig. 28) and to make the first cut with a crude knife.

Transparent "*Scotch*" tape (*Tesa*, Firm of Beiersdorf, Hamburg; *Scotch tape No. 688 or 810* of the Minnesota Mining and Manufacturing Co.) is applied to the smooth section surface with the help of a small brush. The tape must be gently pressed with a brush at the level of the knife edge during passage of the knife (Fig. 30). Before further handling, the section is freeze dried by leaving open in the cryostat for a longer period.

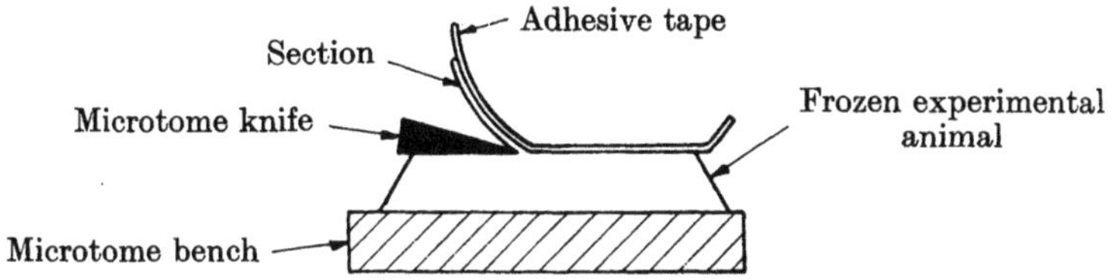

Fig. 30. Diagrammatic representation of the operations in preparing whole-body sections for autoradiography according to ULLBERG

ULLBERG uses *No-screen X-ray Film* for all isotopes except for detecting tritiated substances; he recommends Ilford *G5* plates for these. The dry sections are pressed against the film in the autoradiography. This is therefore a contact procedure, based on the *mounted* method described by EVANS [128] and ENDICOTT and YAGODA [122]. After section and film have been brought into contact, a few sheets of paper are laid on to the rear side of the adhesive tape. The multiple sandwich of paper, tape, section, film or plate and again paper is exposed in a press under slight pressure to ensure that the sandwich holds together without displacement of any part and that contact is even and uniform.

All work with open photographic film material must be performed in indirect safety light, e. g., with the *Kodak Safelight Filter, Wratten No. 6.* The duration of exposure is dictated by the effective activity of the section. A rule of thumb for ^{14}C says that 5 μC per 20 to 25 g body weight (mouse) requires 3 to 4 weeks exposure to give the necessary X-ray film blackening with sections of 20 μ. KALBERER [222] quotes the data in Table 6 for estimating the time of exposure; they refer, however, to his particular experimental conditions.

Table 6

Exposure time for whole-body autoradiography according to KALBERER [222]. The values refer to the X-ray film *Structurix D 10* (Gevaert)

Isotope	Dosage μC/kg	Exposure time in days
^{3}H	10^{4}	30
^{14}C	50	10
^{35}S	50	10
^{59}Fe	100	1

Exposure is carried out in light-tight packing at —20° C. According to the authors, chemographic effects are thereby reduced to a minimum. Film and section are then separated and the film treated as X-ray film. Subsequent treatment of the section (fixation, staining) is always with the tape still adhering. After staining and dehydration in alcohol, section and tape are mounted on a large glass slide or transparent plastic slide and embedded with an alcohol-soluble glue (e. g., *Euparal* from the Firm of Flatters and Garnett, Manchester) under a cover glass.

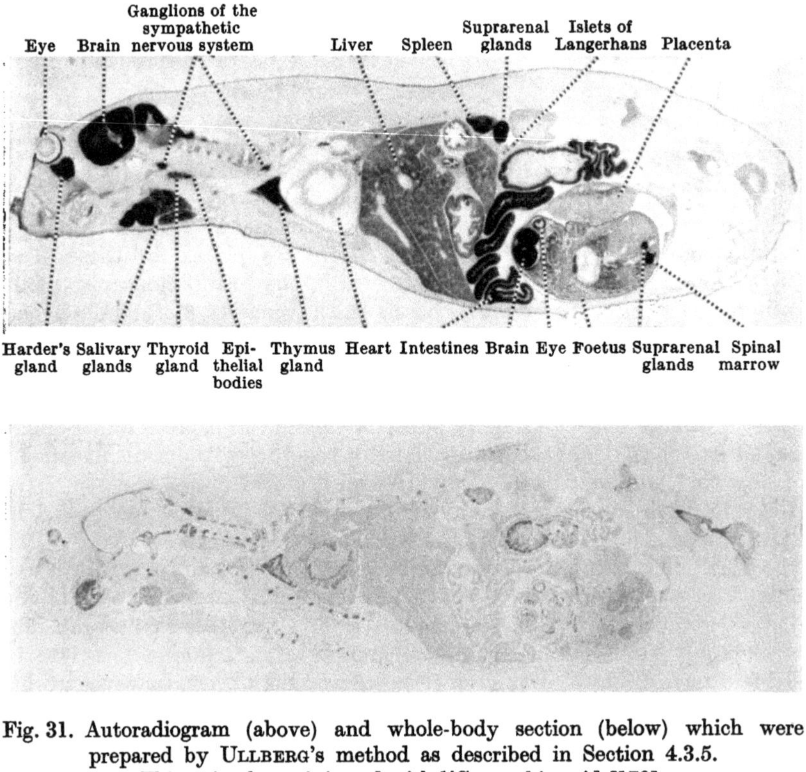

Fig. 31. Autoradiogram (above) and whole-body section (below) which were prepared by ULLBERG's method as described in Section 4.3.5. This animal was injected with ^{14}C-ascorbic acid [179].

4.3.6. Applications of whole-body autoradiography

As has been mentioned already, whole-body autoradiography is utilised in pharmacological investigations: E. g., in surveys of the distribution of pharmaceuticals [116; 117; 339] or their radioactive metabolites; or in observation of the time-dependent uptake in individual organs and tissues. This development has been stimulated by the work of ULLBERG et al in particular [449; 450; 451; 452; 453; 455; 456; 6; 366]. Their investigations include, for instance, studies of the distribution and excretion of penicillin, oestrogens, 5-hydroxytryptamine, 5-hydroxytryptophan and atropine. Next in importance is work on uptake and distribution of inorganic ions or molecules; the toxicological aspect mostly predominated here [116].

An investigation of Sjöstrand, Cassano and Hansson [416] may be cited as an example of pharmacologically slanted whole-body autoradiography: it concerned the distribution of chlorpromazine, a substance with psychotropic activity. Especial interest was centred here on the extent and speed of passage through the blood-brain barrier and through the placenta; and also on the distribution throughout the entire organism. Mice were used as experimental animals. These were injected intravenously with ^{35}S-chlorpromazine (0.25 μC/g body weight). At various intervals after injection, sagittal frozen sections, mostly 20 μ thick, were prepared. The authors observed very high activities in some brain sections already soon after application of the drug. Four hours later there was practically no activity in the brain except in the hippocampus region. The incorporation of activity could be observed also in foetuses. The investigation was even more valuable because the metabolites were characterised chemically in addition. It was possible to demonstrate that, already 20 minutes after injection, the drug had undergone appreciable modification through metabolism. This rendered interpretation of the autoradiograms rather difficult.

The example raises quite generally the question of the usefulness of autoradiography for investigating biological specimens with labelled organic molecules. After all, autoradiography *alone* can elucidate transport routes and regions of sojourn in the living organism for only relatively few substances. These are *non-endogenous* substances which undergo no metabolism. Only for these are the silver grains in the autoradiogram an indicator of their existence in the preparation. In all other cases, silver grains record merely the presence of the particular radioactive *tracer atom*, which may easily belong to any metabolite too. One must emphasise this danger of faulty interpretation of autoradiograms through ignorance of the metabolism of the applied substance. As long as this metabolism is unknown, autoradiograms should be interpreted only to yield negative evidence, e. g., to establish those organ or tissue regions where clearly no incorporation of active material occurs; otherwise, it is possible to speak only of the presence of "radioactive" substance.

The situation is different in autoradiographic studies with inorganic ions, such as phosphate [255] or iodide [454]; the amount present can be established directly from the blackening of the autoradiogram. Naturally, autoradiography gives no information about the nature of the particular chemical bond(s) concerned. Studies on distribution of the sort last mentioned comprise a major part of autoradiographic work so far carried out; they probably exist for almost all elements. Some are of considerable interest in connection with incorporation of radioactive substances which are set free during atomic reactions, such as atom bomb explosions, and which can cause latent radiation damage under certain conditions through their gradual, selective enrichment in definite organs and tissues.

Other whole-body autoradiographic studies concern toxic substances, e. g., mercury compounds. Experiments have been performed with the ^{203}Hg isotope, a relatively powerful β-emitter with a half-life period of only 47 days. Some mercury salts are known to be poorly dissociated in aqueous solution, in contrast to many other inorganic salts which are highly ionised. In these cases, the anionic partner can influence the pharmacological and toxicological properties. Accordingly, autoradiographic investigations on uptake, distribution and elimination of mercury range over a number of different inorganic and organometallic compounds. Examples are mercuric chloride [44], methyl mercuric dicyanodiamide [46] and phenylmercuric acetate [45; 47]. The autoradiograms prepared from each of these substances under comparable conditions show significant differences. Interesting results have been obtained also where both the labelled mercury compound and the known antidote, 2,3-dimercaptopropanol (BAL) were administered [47; 43]. For example, it could be established that accelerated transfer of mercury took place after intravenous injection of methyl ^{203}mercury dicyanodiamide. Moreover, the concentration of mercury in the brain of mice, treated with BAL, was especially high (Fig. 32). Animals treated with the antidote did not show increased mercury elimination. These results cast doubt on the usefulness of BAL in treatment of acute mercury poisoning.

The vexed question of uptake of elementary mercury via the respiratory system does not appear to have been investigated autoradiographically as yet, in contrast to the above work. This is astonishing, since detection of such very small amounts is just the strong point of autoradiography. The same applies to the detection of metallic mercury when inadvertently taken orally.

Further examples of useful application of whole-body autoradiography concern toxic substances, such as pest control agents and herbicides. Thus Bäckström, Hansson and Ullberg [24] investigated metabolic pathways and sites of action of DDT (1,1-p,p'-dichlorodiphenyl-2,2,2-trichloroethane) and dieldrin. Whole-body autoradiography has proved valuable also in studies of rarer elements in the organism, e. g., yttrium [9] or plutonium [456] which can enter the atmosphere after atom bomb explosions and be taken up in traces by the organism via its food*.

* Monographs on the theme "Inhaled Particles and Vapours," by C. N. Davies with many autoradiographic contributions were published by Pergamon Press, N. Y. in 1961 and 1965.

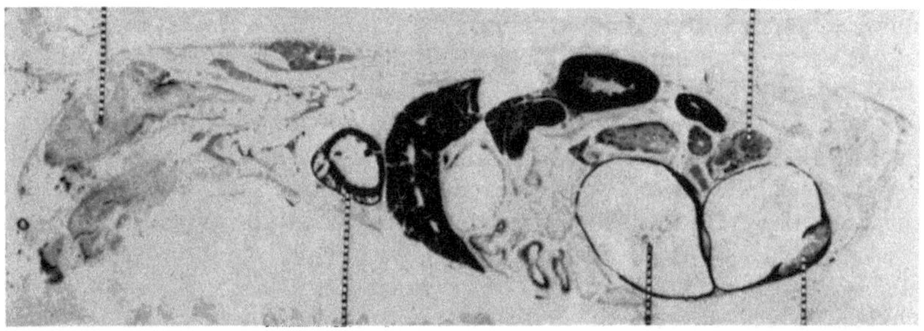

a)

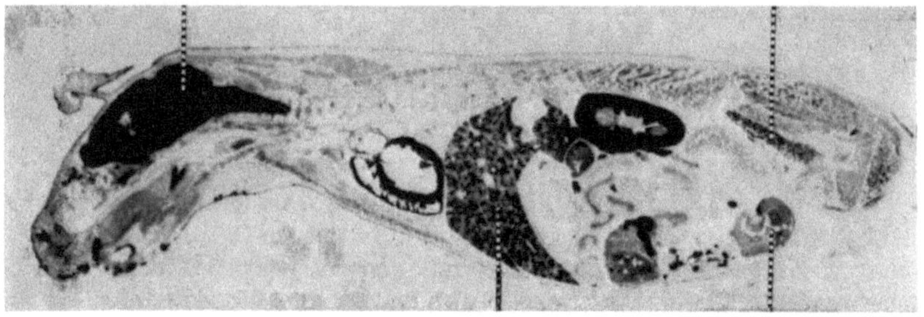

b)

Fig. 32. Autoradiograms of the distribution of ^{203}Hg in sagittal whole-body sections of mice

a) 8 days after injection of phenyl ^{203}mercuric acetate;
b) 8 days after injection of phenyl ^{203}mercuric acetate and BAL. Note the clear differences in uptake between brain and liver of both preparations. From [47]

Reference may be made finally to work by LAL [247] on the distribution of activity of an enzyme. Direct autoradiographic recording of enzymes is practically impossible. Their extracorporal labelling, although in principle not excluded, scarcely achieves the desired end. On account of the difficulty of bringing a labelled enzyme to the site of action in the organism, LAL therefore worked with a type of indirect labelling. He did not label the enzyme under investigation, urease, but used its substrate, urea, in radioactive form. The intensity of blackening of the autoradiogram was regarded as a measure of the enzymatic activity. Evidently this is based on the assumption that substrates or their metabolites concentrate in these areas of higher enzymatic activity. This notion cannot be taken as generally valid for all enzymes or their substrates. LAL based his procedure and the interpretation of the autoradiograms on experiments, likewise evaluated autoradiographically, in which he used inactive substrate and also thiourea, plus free, isolated ureases in place of labelled urea. His autoradiographic pictures of enzyme activity do not conflict with the distribution of urease hitherto known for individual organs and tissues.

The same principle has been extended to microscopic specimens. OSTROWSKI, BARNARD et al [331; 332; 333] investigated autoradiographically the enzymatic activity of acetylcholinesterase in mouse diaphragm, using ^{3}H-diisopropylfluorophosphate as specific inhibitor. In reference studies with acetylthiocholine, with which the motor endplates can be selectively stained, it could be proved that the autoradiographic blackening was strictly limited to the endplates. The same subject has been treated by SALPETER, ROGERS and BARNARD [393] in an electron-microscopic autoradiographic study.

4.4. Other macroscopic specimens

4.4.1. Distribution of iron in magnetic recording tapes

The quality of reproduction of sound recordings on magnetic tapes depends on the homogeneity of distribution of the magnetisable material, amongst other factors. This material is usually a mixture of Fe(II) and Fe(III) oxides. MAKIN and NUNLEY [281] developed a method for checking this distribution of magnetisable material in recording tapes. The iron, which occurs in nature as a mixture of isotopes, is converted by neutron bombardment (see Section 4.1.1., Table 2) into the isotopes ^{57}Fe and ^{58}Fe, predominantly β-emitters. The authors submitted samples of sound tape for a period of 5 days to a flux of about 10^{12} neutrons/cm^2/sec. After this neutron activation, the samples were placed against *Kodaline* Film (Kodak) for an exposure period of ca 24 hours.

The material under investigation was especially suited to neutron activation since it had a relatively high iron content. Examination of the non-ferrous radioactive products was, however, essential. The authors made use of autoradiograms of various samples which had been subjected to different periods of neutron activation; and also of the analysis of the γ-ray spectrum of the activated sound tape samples and of the times of decay of activity. They were then able to show that, under the given experimental conditions, scarcely any other emitters were present which could falsify the autoradiographic reproduction of iron distribution to an extent worth mentioning.

Both macroscopic and microscopic irregularities were noted in the distribution of iron in the sound tape material. Those 1 to 3 mm apart could be seen even with the naked eye (Fig. 33a). Inhomogeneities in the 5 μ region were visible in the microscope (Fig. 33b) and were clearly due to fluctuations in the iron distribution.

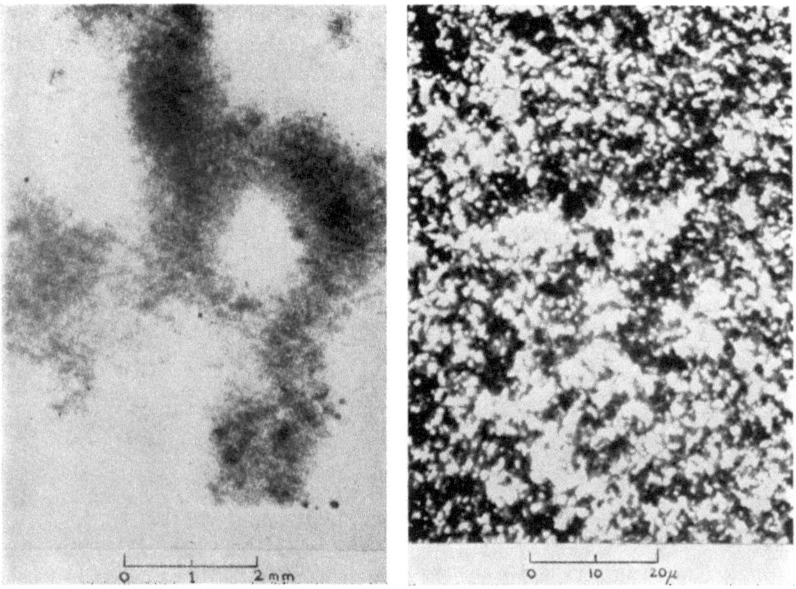

a) b)

Fig. 33. Distribution of iron in magnetic sound tapes, according to MAKIN and NUNLEY [281]

a) macroscopic; b) microscopic inhomogeneities

4.4.2. Criminological study of handwritten documents

GORDON and LISICHENKO [161] described a method of detection of alterations to documents, important in criminology. It permits location of all changes carried out with ink of chemical composition different from that used in the original. Even forgeries with the same ink can be detected if the original is appreciably older than that used in the alteration.

The part of the document being investigated is soaked with a 0.1 N silver nitrate solution, acidified with nitric acid and containing 1 mC ^{110}Ag/ml; or with a thallium sulphate solution which contains ^{204}Tl. After 5 minutes, excess reagent is washed out with 0.01% nitric acid. The piece of document in dried and stored in darkness in close contact with photographic paper. This paper is developed in the usual way about 24 hours later.

This method is more sensitive than any purely chemical analytical method for testing documents. It depends on the radioactive tracer combining with components, chiefly chloride ions, of the dried out ink. The salts formed are poorly soluble and thus remain on the paper. Aniline dyes, constituents of many inks, also adsorb silver and thallium ions although they contain negligible amounts of chloride ion. Handwriting of this sort is therefore radioactively labelled also. The authors were able to show that the extent of adsorption of silver is determined by the age of the writing (Fig. 34). The degree of adsorption of basic dyes for silver and thallium ions is independent of the age of the writing, in contrast to the findings with acid dyes.

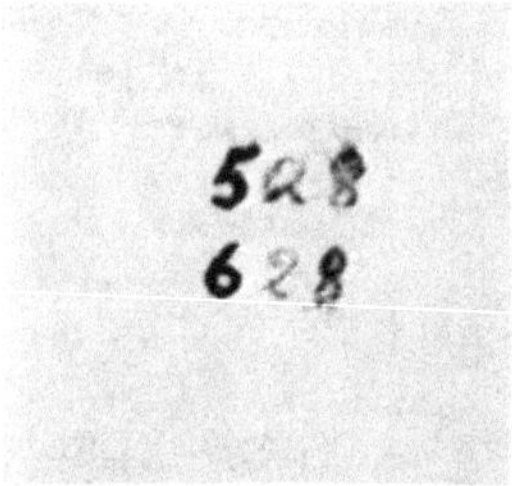

Fig. 34. From GORDON and LISICHENKO [161]
Autoradiogram of a sample of writing with methyl violet ink, after treatment with an acidic $^{110}AgNO_3$ solution. The figures "5" and "6" were added with the same ink eighteen months after the main text, with the figures "28," had been written. The alteration is first recognisable in the autoradiogram

GORDON and LISICHENKO worked also with complex anions, such as $[Fe(CN)_6]^{4-}$, $[Zn(SCN)_4]^{2-}$, $[TlBr_4]^-$ and $[CdI_4]^{2-}$. They found distinct differences in autoradiographic blackening when using these ions, tagged with ^{35}S, ^{131}I or ^{14}C. These differences were in agreement with the rule of Fajans and Paneth, that the ion yielding the least soluble product with the dye is that which is most strongly adsorbed. It is therefore possible to distinguish between writing with ink of the same colour but of different make (Fig. 35). The procedure is said to be useful also to detect forgeries with inks used for stamping.

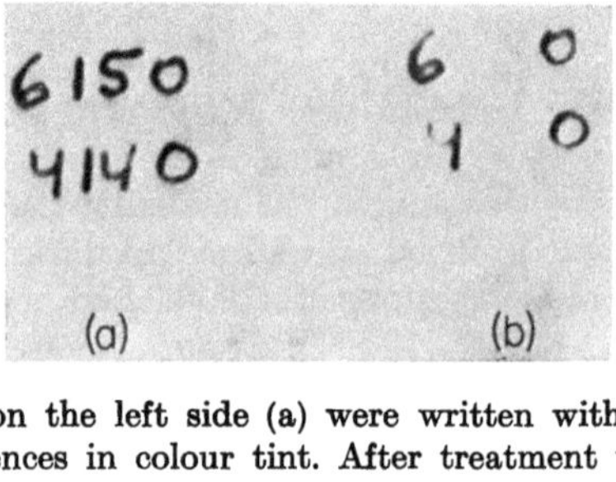

Fig. 35. The figures on the left side (a) were written with methylene blue ink. They show no differences in colour tint. After treatment with potassium ferrocyanide (^{14}C), the autoradiogram of these figures (b) reveals that different inks have been used. From GORDON and LISICHENKO [161]

4.4.3. Detection of fingerprints

The usual methods for detecting and visualising fingerprints fail when they are on paper and textiles. TAKEUCHI, SAKAGUCHI and NAKAMOTO [436] worked out a procedure which eliminates this weakness in day to day criminological investigation. It permits detection and recording of latent fingerprints on paper, wood and textile material (except silk and wool).

This autoradiographic procedure for fingerprint detection is based on the affinity of formaldehyde vapour for skin secretions (e. g. amino acids or amines) which are always present in traces on handled objects and which delineate the papillae. The procedure is roughly as follows: Radioactively labelled formaldehyde (commercially available, for example, as ^{14}C-paraformaldehyde) is treated with sulphuric acid and introduced into an evacuated glass vessel (200 ml at 20 mm pressure). This is connected via a valve to another glass vessel which contains the sample. This vessel is exposed to light from a lamp for about 10 minutes to accelerate the reaction. Excess aldehyde is then drawn off, the samples are aerated and taken out of the reaction vessel. The positions of suspected fingerprints are tested with a Geiger-Muller counter and fingerprints localised. The areas identified in this way can be brought into contact with X-ray film in a darkroom with suitable safelighting. Sample and film are then stored together at + 5°C in a dry atmosphere in total darkness. The time of exposure can be estimated from the activity measured with the counter. A reading of 6 to 8 impulses/cm^2 yields a good fingerprint autoradiogram already in 24 hours. Clearer pictures are obtained when the samples are briefly rinsed with water before

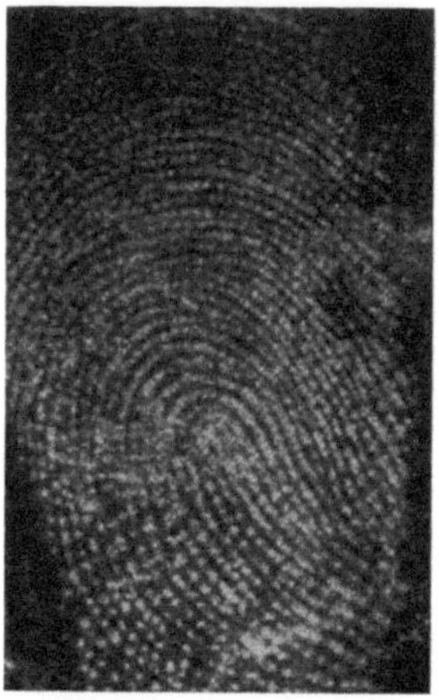

Fig. 36. Autoradiogram of a fingerprint on paper according to TAKEUCHI, SAKAGUCHI and NAKAMOTO [436]

exposure with the film; this removes excess, loosely adsorbed aldehyde. Lelenthal and Szuchnik [256] give other procedures for autoradiographic detection of fingerprints.

4.4.4. Dispersion of fillers in rubber

Fillers are used in preparing rubber articles, especially tyres, in order to impart a quality to the product suited to its expected treatment. Grain size and distribution of filler play significant parts in this. For instance, the tensile strength of products increases with the degree of distribution of filler (for the same starting material composition). A homogeneous distribution of the filler is the usual target.

Kirshenbaum et al [230] studied autoradiographically the dependence of the dispersion of carbon, added as carbon black to rubber, on the nature and duration of the mixing and milling processes used in rubber production. The filler had to be labelled without influencing the normal grain size distribution. This was accomplished with the apparatus depicted in Fig. 37. 25 g carbon black were placed in the quartz tube 3 and degassed by heating at 1000° C and pumping off all the desorbed gases. 35 mg $Ba^{14}CO_3$ (0.5 mC) were treated with phosphoric acid in the decomposition tube A. The $^{14}CO_2$ liberated was dried in the cool trap 1 and condensed in trap 2 with the help of liquid nitrogen. It was distilled into

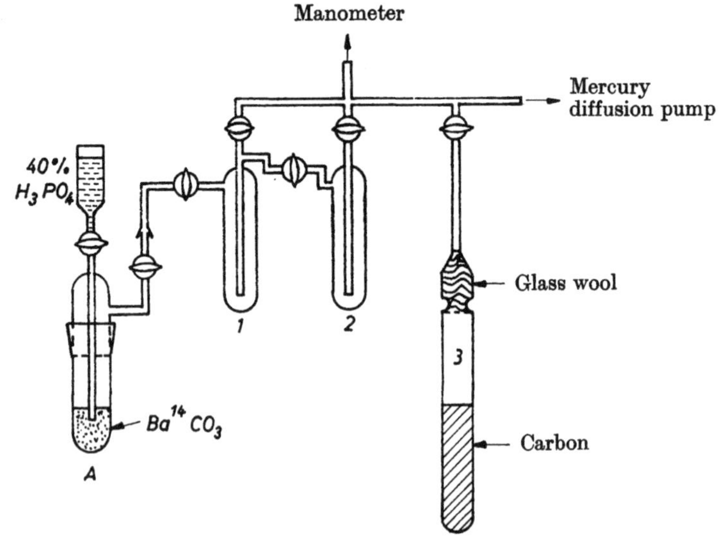

Fig. 37. Apparatus for preparing ^{14}C from $Ba^{14}CO_3$, according to Kirshenbaum et al [230]. See text for details

the quartz vessel 3 where it reacted with the carbon black at 900—1000° C according to the equation,

$$C + {}^{14}CO_2 \rightleftharpoons {}^{14}C + 2CO.$$

Since the carbon black was in enormous excess of the amount of carbon in the radioactive carbon dioxide, only a trace of the radioactivity introduced could be detected in the gas phase after $5^1/_2$ hours reaction. The grain size distribution of the radioactive filler should not be modified by this procedure. The filler was diluted with inactive material and mixed until the activity distribution was homogeneous. It was then used directly in the production process.

Flat rubber strips about 2.5 cm broad were used for preparing the autoradiograms. After exposure with X-ray film for 3 days, using ordinary

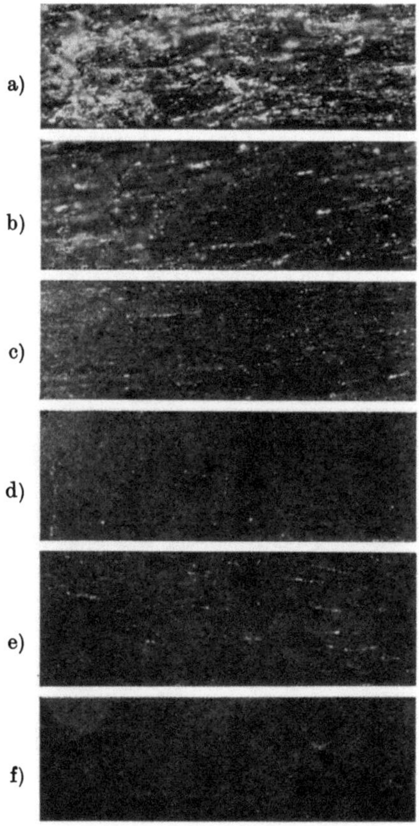

Fig. 38. Contact autoradiograms of some rubber samples with labelled filler, according to KIRSHENBAUM et al [230]. The degree of dispersion of the filler diminishes from a) to f)

printing frames from photographic laboratories, development and fixing were carried out. Fig. 38 shows some autoradiograms of rubber samples with various filler dispersions, prepared in this way. The authors report a far better differentiation of filler dispersion using the autoradiographic method than microscopically with sections of 10 μ thickness; this is possible even when the material appears homogeneous in the microscope.

Herrmann, Hartmann, Bothe and Hofmann [188] describe a procedure for studying dispersion of silicic acid filler in rubber which may be given as an example of labelling through ion adsorption, seldom encountered: Samples of 1 cm cross-section were punched out of industrially prepared rubber slabs, carefully cleaned and immersed for two days in a dilute aqueous solution of ^{32}P-labelled K_2HPO_4 of specific activity 0.1 mC/ml. The adhering radioactive solution was then washed off and the samples covered with a thin film of the plastic emulsion, *Mowital*. (Blank experiments had shown that inactive rubber can blacken photographic emulsion; this effect was not mentioned by Kirshenbaum et al [230].

Labelling by ion adsorption was chosen since it is not possible to label the silicic acid (e. g. with ^{32}Si) directly in the normal production process on account of the high activities needed. It was expected of the rubber-filler system that the rubber itself would not adsorb phosphate ions anything like as strongly as the silicic acid filler. The authors report direct measurements of activity on rubber with various contents of silicic acid filler. They found that activity increased roughly exponentially with filler content of the samples. It is evident from this that lumps of filler should show up especially strongly in the autoradiograms. Figs 39a and b show autoradiograms obtained after exposure for several

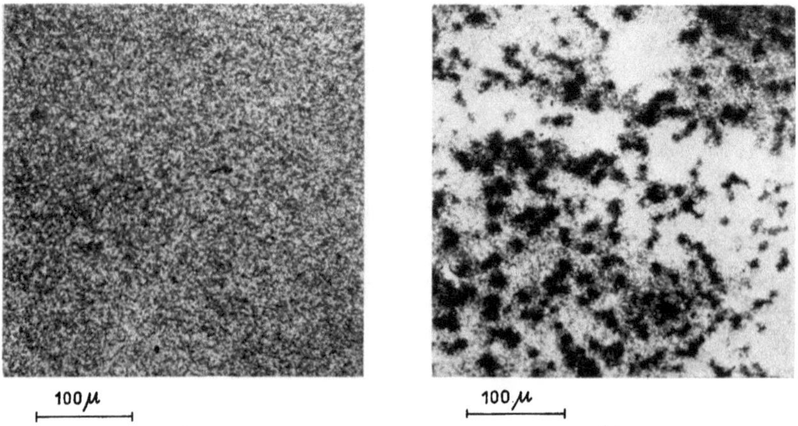

a) b)

Fig. 39. Autoradiograms of silicic acid filler in rubber, according to Herrmann et al [188]. Labelling was performed by ion adsorption of $K_2H^{32}PO_4$

a) homogeneous; b) inhomogeneous distribution

days of film (*Kernspurplatte K2* or *Strippingfilm K 102* of VEB Agfa-Wolfen, GDR) pressed moderately fimly against suitably even sample surfaces. Development was shortened in order to increase definition. Only those layers of the relatively thick emulsion nearest to the sample were developed and not the more deeply-seated layers. The blackening of these latter would have impaired the quality of the autoradiogram as a result of the great range and scattering of the radiation.

4.4.5. Investigations of transport of material in soil samples

JOHNSTON [219] studied the influence of rainwater on the transport of minerals in soil samples. He filled soil into transparent plastic tubes which had been halved along their lengths. The two halves were held together with a second, enveloping tube made of the same material. The internal diameter of the part containing the soil samples was about 6 cm. Various sets of experimental conditions could be tested with this equipment and natural soil-water conditions simulated. The dependence of the transport of a mineral substance (e. g. a manurial salt) on the amount of rainwater could be followed by freezing individual columns in dry ice at appropriate times. The enclosing tube was then removed and the filling cut up with a band saw. Brushes pressed against the rotating saw blade removed from it adhering sawdust which would otherwise have contaminated the cut surface. The autoradiograms were prepared by the contact procedure. Exposure had to be carried out at temperatures below 0° C since the frozen soil samples would otherwise have thawed and displacement could have occurred. A thin (5 μ) film of plastic on the surface served as protection against chemography. SÜSS [435] and DATTA and SRIVASTAVA [90] have described similar equipment for autoradiography of soil samples.

4.5. Specimens with irregularly shaped surfaces

Irregular specimens create technical difficulties. Neither the stripping film technique (Section 5.1.) nor contact autoradiography (Chapter 4.) can be employed since they require specimens with plane surfaces. Primarily only those methods can be considered where a suitable surface coating is obtained through dipping the specimen into a liquid photographic emulsion, so that enough emulsion remains adhering to the uneven surface. A condition of this "*dipping*" technique is that chemography does not occur. Otherwise, the surface must be previously treated with an inert varnish or spray of synthetic plastic. "*Stripping*" type procedures can nevertheless be used and the examples below show how difficultly accessible cavities can be studied autoradiographically with the help of various artifices.

4.5.1. Autoradiograms of the surfaces of bones, shells and similar solid bodies

JODREY and WILBUR [214] in their investigations of the formation of mollusc shells faced the problem of determining autoradiographically the incorporation and distribution of ^{45}Ca- and ^{32}P-compounds in the inner walls of mussels. The simplest procedure, that of immersing the specimens in a liquid emulsion, was expected to yield insufficiently uniformly coated surfaces. This would have sufficed for qualitative studies but not, however, for the quantitative work planned (Section 7.1.). Consequently the decision was taken to adopt a method based on the stripping procedure (Section 5.1.) of X-ray film (*Eastman Industrial X-ray Film, Type A*); the emulsion layer was to be detached and stuck in strips on to the surface of the specimen. Pieces of X-ray film corresponding to the size of the specimens, were first soaked for 5 minutes in water at 30° C. The radiation-sensitive gelatine layer was carefully

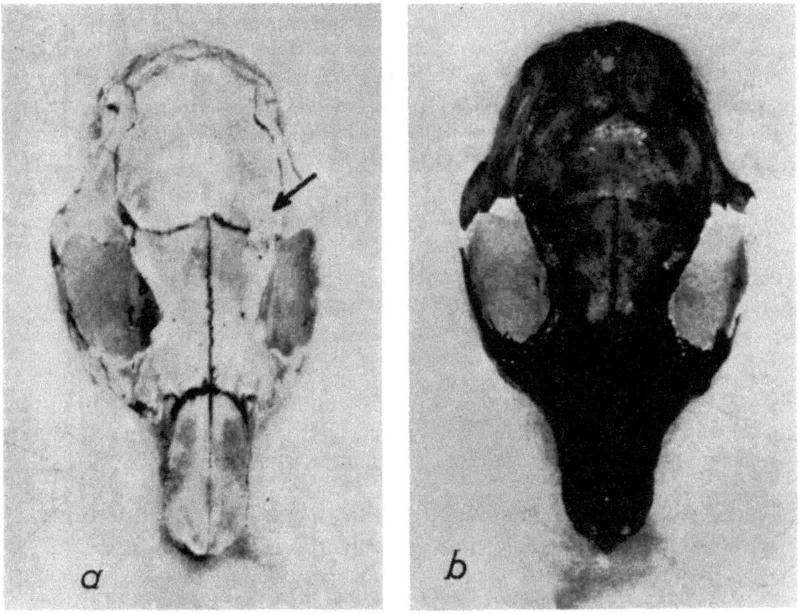

Fig. 40. Autoradiograms from JODREY and WILBUR [214]

a) Even a skull of a guinea pig without injection of radioactive material shows intense blackening at some cranial sutures. The immediate vicinity of the sutures cannot therefore be studied with this method. The skull bone was removed in the vicinity of the arrow.

b) Autoradiogram of a guinea pig skull. The animal received 100 μC ^{32}P (presumably as phosphate) applied intraperitoneally 20 hours before killing. Time of exposure: 1 day. Clear differences in blackening are recognisable

loosened at one corner from the carrier with the edge of a glass slide; the carrier was then completely detached. The specimens were brought up from below to the pieces of emulsion layer, floating in the water, in such a way that on lifting out of the water bath, the radiation-sensitive layer came in contact with those parts of the specimens to be autoradiographed. The soaked plastic film clings fairly tenaciously to the profile of the specimen. If necessary, it can be gently pressed on with a soft, moistened brush.
The procedure is suitable for bone surfaces also (Fig. 40).

4.5.2. *In vivo*-autoradiography of internal body surfaces

It has long been known that tumour tissue takes up phosphates in increased amounts. As early as 1949, SELVERSTONE and co-workers [405] detected brain tumours through their enriched concentration of ^{32}P. Similar experiments were carried out later in connection with cancerous tumours of the oesophagus and the stomach [318]. The method has the disadvantage of limited clinical applicability: radiation from ^{32}P has a range of only about 1 cm, so that precise localisation of the sites concerned did not appear possible. On the other hand, *in vitro*-autoradiography of resected organs yielded good topographical pictures of the extent of pathological change. ACKERMAN, SHAHON, MCFEE and WANGENSTEEN [3; 406] subsequently engaged in a study of *in vivo*-autoradiography of the stomach.
The method which they developed [2] has an original principle. An ordinary rubber contraceptive was first coated on the outside with a special elastic photographic emulsion (*Kodak Autoradiographic Elastic Film, Type 1*). After the emulsion had dried, the contraceptive was turned inside out so that the radiation-sensitive layer was on the inside. A stomach tube containing two separate canals was attached to the open end (Fig. 41). The whole system was introduced into the patient's stomach via the nose. On the previous day the patient had received an injection of 500 μC ^{32}P as sodium phosphate. About 100 ml air were first blown into the contraceptive balloon. Subsequent operations could be carried out in normal illumination since there was no further danger of exposure to light. Secretion products were sucked through the second canal of the stomach tube from the patient in a lying position. The balloon was then filled with 200 ml air and forced deeply into the stomach until a distinct resistance was felt; its upper end is then at the oesophagus. This fixation is important for the subsequent topographical evaluation of the autoradiogram. Further air was then blown into the contraceptive until it had expanded to a maximum of ca 1 litre content. After exposure of several hours, the air was allowed to escape and the balloon removed in the dark room. It was rubbed over with glycerine and pulled over a

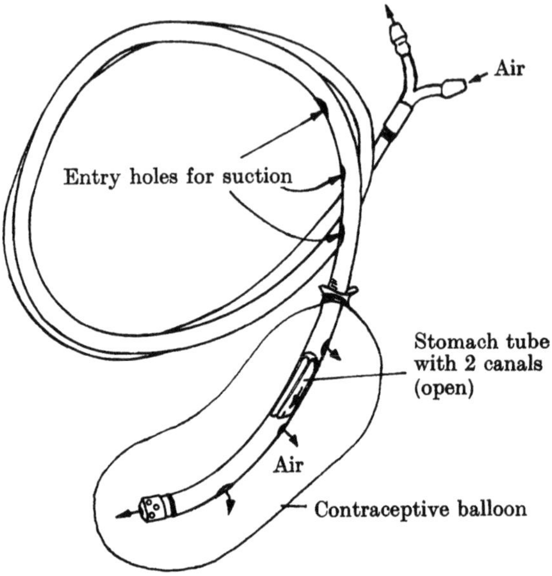

Fig. 41. Contraceptive-balloon autoradiography with stomach tube. According to Ackerman, McFee and Wangensteen [2]. Explanatory details in text

suitably sized test tube so that the emulsion was outside again. This assisted photographic development and subsequent handling.
The autoradiogram shows blackening on all sites with neoplasm, which can be evaluated diagnostically (Fig. 42).
It might be expected that the wall of the inflated contraceptive balloon would offer no special resistance to the β-radiation of ^{32}P. A comparison of various materials showed that the polyurethane, *Vithane*, permits about 3 to 4 times shorter exposure time than Latex rubber and must therefore possess a very low β-absorption coefficient (Section 7.4.).

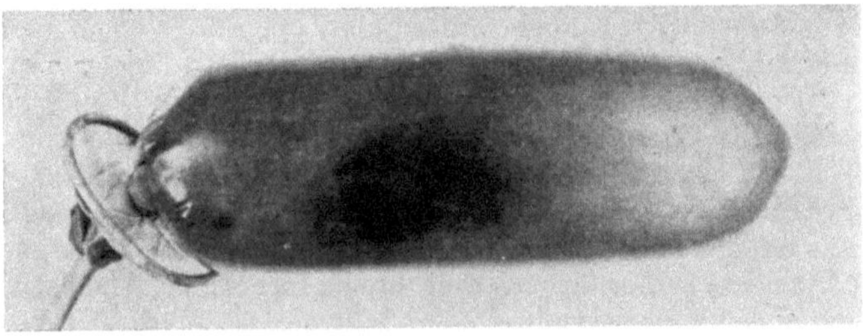

Fig. 42. *In vivo* contraceptive-balloon autoradiogram of the stomach with intense blackening due to a carcinoma. From [3]. Explanatory details in text

5. AUTORADIOGRAPHY OF MICROSCOPIC SPECIMENS

5.1. General

In the present chapter the autoradiography of those specimens is treated which cannot be distinguished with the naked eye. This includes studies of bacteria or protozoa and also larger preparations where the detection of radioactivity in microscopic structures is of interest. In contrast to the autoradiography of larger specimens, treated above, interest is focussed here on the precision of identification of the radiation sites in the preparation which are responsible for blackening in the autoradiogram. All autoradiographic techniques discussed above in connection with larger specimens have been applied in principle to microscopically small specimens as well. One encounters thus: 1. *Contact methods* (*apposition technique*) in which specimen and photographic layer are separated after exposure and then further treated separately. 2. Techniques with permanent contact between preparation and film. The *stripping film procedure* belongs to these, in which ready prepared sheets of film are used; and also methods based on the use of so-called liquid emulsions. These last named include the *mounting procedure* (the sections of tissue under investigation are stuck directly to a prepared photoemulsion) and its converse, the *coating technique* (the radiation-sensitive layer is brought on to the prepared histological sections, either as drops of a diluted emulsion which are then spread over the surface; or by briefly immersing the specimen in an emulsion of suitable consistency — the *dipping procedure*)

There are many variants of these procedures. Only those techniques are treated below which have attained greater importance.

5.2. Stripping film autoradiography

5.2.1. Technique

Since its introduction by Pelc [342, 344], MacDonald, Cobbs, Solomon and Steinberg [279] and Berriman, Herz and Stevens [48], the stripping film procedure has been that most widely used in autoradiography. This is probably because commercially available film material can be employed. This possesses the advantages of relatively easy handling; of almost universal applicability to practically all radioisotopes of interest in histochemistry; and of comparatively high sensitivity to radiation and good contact with the preparation.

Stripping films consist of a nuclear emulsion layer, attached firmly to a layer of gelatine. The film *AR 10* (Kodak), the prototype of all stripping films, is 15 μ thick, only 4 μ of which constitute the real emulsion layer. The film is marketed on glass plates for reasons of stability. The gelatine layer is in direct contact with the glass. The term *stripping film* is derived from the custom of peeling off pieces of film of desired sizes from this glass support. The pieces are first cut around with a sharp knife. For manufacturing and packing reasons, a margin of about 0.5 cm around the 12 × 16.5 cm *AR 10* plates is not suitable for autoradiography. The dry stripped pieces are laid with the emulsion layer below on the surface of water at room temperature in a water bath. The

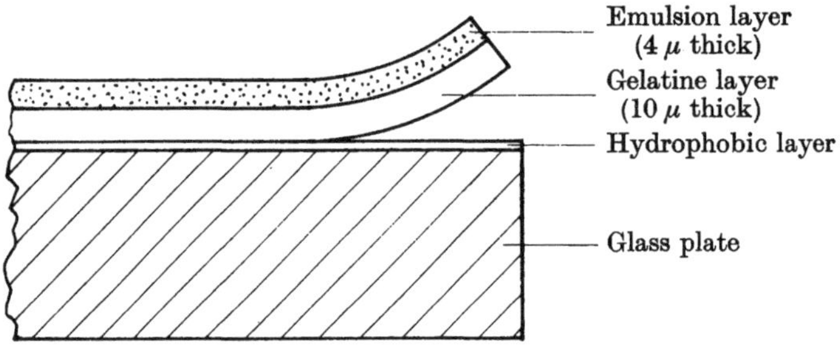

Fig. 43. Section through a commercial stripping film (schematic)

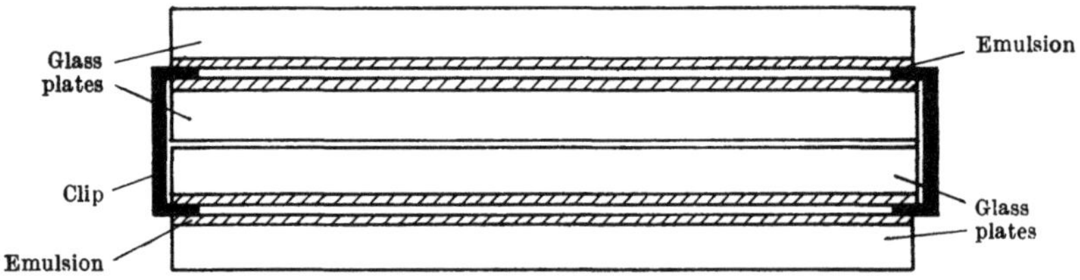

Fig. 44. For marketing, stripping films are packed in the way illustrated schematically here, in order to protect the film layer. A plastic clip spaces them suitably

stripping film imbibes water and swells to its maximum size in about 3 to 5 minutes without sinking. The stripping film is most conveniently applied to the specimen when the latter is on a glass slide. This applies practically always to histological preparations which are in the form of thin sections.

The glass slide is best covered with a gelatine layer in order to achieve maximum adhesion of preparation to stripping film. The slides are cleaned in dilute chromic acid/sulphuric acid for this purpose. The glass surface is "clean" when it can be wetted uniformly with a film of water. The well-rinsed and cleaned slides are then dipped into the solution:

5.0 g gelatine
0.5 g chrome alum
water up to 1 litre

and finally air dried without rinsing.
The stripping film is "fished" from the surface of the water using the gelatine-covered glass slides, so that the radiation-sensitive layer is deposited on the preparation. Any overlapping film is folded round the edge of the slide (Fig. 45). The coated preparations are dried by storing horizontally in the air for about 2 hours. The relative humidity should be 60—70%. If the air is not moist enough, the film may become detached from the specimen or electrostatic potential differences may become established between film and preparation glass, which can lead to exposure of the film [169; 299]. Incidentally, this can occur when the film is detached too rapidly from the glass carrier plate on which it is supplied. Under dry conditions, even sparks may be observed. All operations with stripping film must naturally be conducted in a dark room with safelighting. The *Kodak Safelight Filter Wratten 1* with a maximum of 25 watts is recommended for the film material *AR 10*. Even then, as little light as possible should fall on the film. Unused stripping film material can be stored in the original packing for up to 6 months at temperatures below + 20° C. Parallel considerations apply to the autoradiographic exposure. No generalisation can be made, of course, about the time neces-

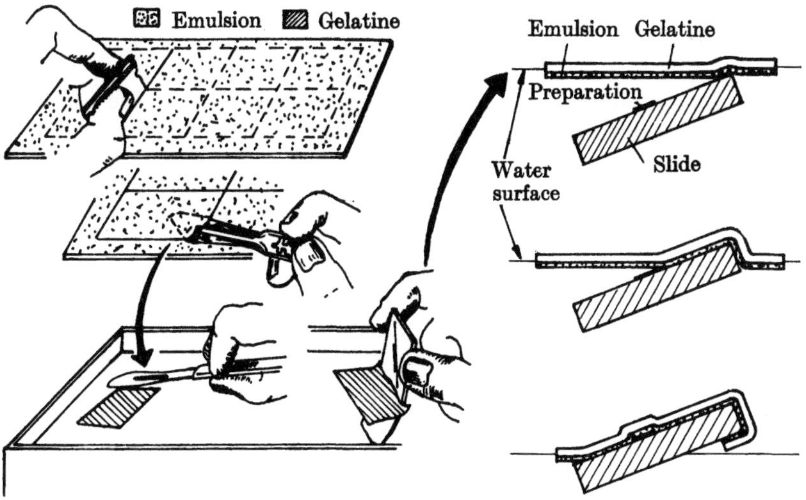

Fig. 45. Schematic representation of the application of stripping film. See text for details

sary for exposure. This depends on the nature of the emitter used, its concentration and the mechanical character of the preparation. As a rough rule, 10 μ sections with an activity of 1 μC/ml tissue require an exposure of at least 14 days.

The developers *D 19* or *D 19b* (Kodak) are recommended (Tab. 7) for development, using a time of up to 30 minutes. The development process has practically concluded after 5—10 minutes. After halting development by briefly washing with water (30 seconds), fixing is carried out in the Kodak fixing bath *F 5*; the fixing time is twice that needed for the initially cloudy film to become fully clear. After rinsing for 1 hour in running water, the stripping film autoradiograms are placed horizontally and dried in dust-free air.

Table 7

Composition of the developer *D 19b* (Kodak)

p-Methylaminophenol sulphate ('metol,' 'elon')	2.2 g
Sodium sulphite (anhydrous)	72 g
(or $Na_2SO_3 \cdot 7H_2O$)	144 g
Hydroquinone	8.8 g
Sodium carbonate, anhydrous	48 g
(or $Na_2CO_3 \cdot 10H_2O$)	130 g
Potassium bromide	4.0 g

The compounds are dissolved in water in the order quoted and the volume of solution made up to 1 litre.

Stripping films other than the *AR 10* are marketed; these are, however, comparatively seldom used. Whereas *AR 10* emulsion has an average silver halide grain diameter of about 0.2 μ, the Kodak stripping film *AR 50* has a larger average grain diameter and the emulsion layer is about 12 μ thick. The larger grain diameter yields a higher sensitivity to radiation. The autoradiographic resolution with *AR 50* is too inferior for histological purposes. This type of film is considered primarily for macroscopic specimens although at the present time there is still a preference for contact procedures with X-ray films that are easier to handle. The *Kodak stripping film V1062* is commercially available; it has the same emulsion and emulsion layer thickness as the *AR 10* but has no supporting gelatine layer. This material was evolved for autoradiography of preparations labelled with two isotopes. It is first exposed and then developed; the autoradiogram obtained is covered again with stripping film and once more exposed and developed. This second exposure is to detect that labelled material with radiation of higher energy and range, which passes through the first autoradiogram; it yields a second autoradiogram with the second film layer when a suitably long time of exposure is chosen. This procedure is described by FIELD, DAWSON and STEVENS [133] and FIELD, DAWSON and GIBBS [132] for differentiating material tagged with both ^{3}H and ^{14}C. It has not enjoyed extensive application, probably because double labelling is relatively rarely undertaken.

The film *V1062* should have a slight advantage over *AR 10* in that the possibilities of staining the preparation are less restricted as a result of the thinner covering by the photographic layer.

The same firm provides also special products which differ from stripping film *AR 10* in having still thinner emulsion layers (down to 1μ). This material was created with the aim of still better autoradiographic resolution, yet finds only sporadic application. There is no proof that resolution really is improved with such especially thin stripping films. It appears that reduction of the thickness of the emulsion beyond a certain value brings no additional benefit; resolution does not depend alone on the thickness of the film layer.

Little has been published about the use of stripping films of the firm of Ilford. VEB Agfa Wolfen (GDR) also prepare stripping films, of which *K 102* and *K 105* have proved valuable in metal autoradiography [459]. These last mentioned films are handled as described for *AR 10*.

5.2.2. Examples

It is impossible to make even an approximate list of all the many applications of stripping films. They are used above all in problems of biology and medicine. The two following examples, which are representative of many similar successful applications, may demonstrate at least the efficiency of the stripping film method in the autoradiography of microscopically small biological specimens.

Fig. 46 shows the extremely high resolution of a chromosome autoradiogram. DENNIS and WAKE [96] isolated chromosomes from *Bacillus subtilis*, cultures of which had grown for about two generations on a culture medium containing ^{3}H-thymidine. As a result of their high thymidine content, the chromosomes appear in the autoradiogram as thread-like forms over their entire lengths.

The next example illustrates the high sensitivity of stripping film autoradiography which enables autoradiograms to be obtained of mice to which less than 1 μg of a labelled substance had been previously administered.

The paralysing effect of the Indian arrow poison, curare, has been the object of detailed pharmacological studies for over 100 years. The result of these is the recognition of the motor endplates as the probable site of action of the curare, i. e., the points of attachment of nerves to skeletal muscles. Investigations on, and direct evidence about, the whereabouts of curare-like substances in the organism appeared impossible for a long time, since the amounts of active compounds are minute. The site of activity of this substance was first directly located with

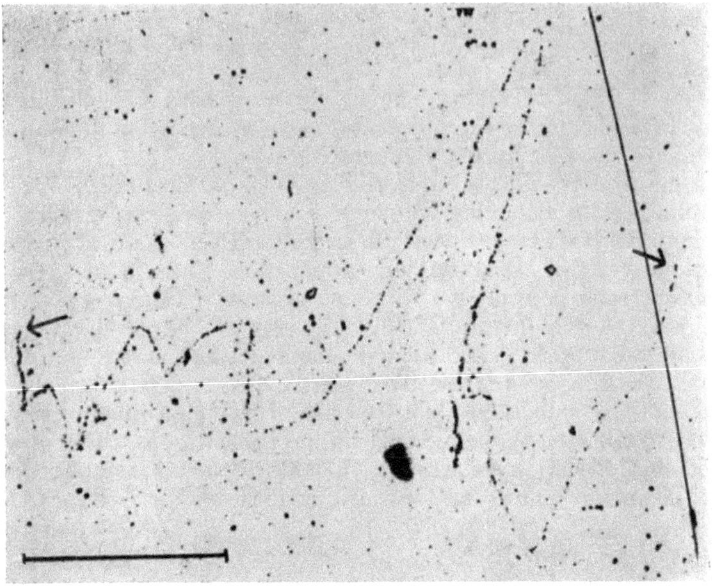

Fig. 46. Autoradiogram of an intact, uncoiled chromosome from *B. subtilis*. Labelled through addition of tritiated thymidine in the culture medium of the rapidly growing cells. The ends of the chromosome are denoted by arrows. The drawn-in horizontal line represents 100 μ on the scale used. From [96]

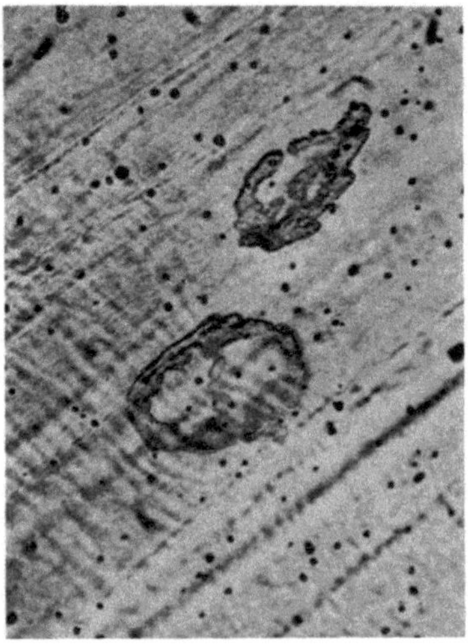

Fig. 47. Endplates of the diaphragm of a mouse after dosage with 0.22 μg ^{14}C-curarine. Autoradiogram with stripping film *AR 10*. Time of exposure of 60 days. Magnification ca 1,000x. From [463]

the help of isotope labelling in combination with autoradiography [462; 463; 464]. *Calabash-curarine* I with relatively high specific activity (24 μC/mg) was first synthesised. Minimum lethal doses (0.22 μg) were injected intravenously into mice. Contact autoradiograms with X-ray film of the immediately sampled diaphragms showed an activity enrichment in the region of the endplates. Only when the stripping film technique was employed could a concentration of activity over the endplates themselves be demonstrated (Fig. 47).
The number of curarine molecules per endplate was calculated approximately to obtain information on at least the order of occupation of the surfaces of the receptors when all synapses are completely blocked. This yielded a result of ca 8.10^6 molecules curarine bound to one endplate. The resolution of the autoradiogram was, however, insufficient to permit localisation of the radioactivity to a particular structure in the endplate. The competitive antagonism to acetylcholine, known from other experiments, renders it probable that the cholinergic receptors of the subneural layer are occupied with curare.

5.2.3. Advantages and limitations

As has already been mentioned, the Kodak film *AR 10* is the most commonly used stripping flim, so that assessment of the stripping film procedure is based mainly on experience gained with this film. There are various reasons for this popularity of the stripping film: a relatively easily adaptable technique; and the nature and properties of the film material itself.
It may be said basically that stripping film is absolutely the most suitable autoradiographic film material for all laboratories in which autoradiography is occasionally used along with chemical-analytical or other methods to solve particular problems.
The thickness of the emulsion layer, the size of the silver halide crystals, the grain distribution and sensitivity to radiation of stripping film are always constant as a result of standardised manufacture. This film thus fulfils all requirements for reproducible qualitative and quantitative work. Further, the relatively high sensitivity over a wide range of radiation energy, scarcely attainable with liquid emulsions, favours the choice of stripping film [85]. Both α- and β-emitters can be detected with the same material. The autoradiographic resolution with microscopic specimens can scarcely be bettered (see Section 5.2.4.). It is stated that silver grains can be coordinated with specimen details of only 1 μ diameter. Evaluation is on the whole facilitated by the fact that the film adheres directly to the specimen.
In other respects, however, the stripping film method can possess disadvantages. Firstly, one must mention the stripping procedure, described in detail in Section 5.2.1. From the separation of the film from carrier

plate right up to the drying stage, with all its requirements concerning air humidity and manual dexterity, it is most demanding compared to other methods, as far as they are pursued in routine work. The permanent attachment of photographic layer to preparation can also be a problem. This applies especially to the indispensable staining procedure in histoautoradiography, which can suffer serious interference from the firmly adhering photographic layer and from the gelatine carrier layer which adsorbs the dye. Only slight improvement is achieved if stripping film without gelatine carrier is employed, because the film gelatine also can adsorb dyes. The suggestion has repeatedly been made of staining histological sections before the stripping film is applied [84]. But it is then necessary to check whether the staining procedure affects the autoradiography. Positive chemography has sometimes been observed after histological staining. For example DEUCHAR [100] found a general increase in the silver grain background after staining with Celestine Blue. Staining of histological preparations before their autoradiographic exposure may cause problems even when there is no chemography. Radioactively labelled substances may be dissolved or displaced [223; 252]. Worthy of note in this connection is an observation of STÖCKER and MÜLLER [430] that stripping film autoradiography is equally incompatible with the orcein-pressing method, used in the more modern cytology. They made "pseudo-autoradiograms" from non-radioactive preparations which had been previously stained with orcein; they found silver grains corresponding to numerous cell nuclei, already after 24 hours "exposure". There was evidently a direct relation between the local adsorption of the staining dye in the chromocentres of liver cell nuclei, which form especially compact heterochromatic nuclear structures, and the particular local density of silver grain (Fig. 48). In other respects, however, the description in Section 5.3. of histological staining reactions when liquid emulsions are used, applies likewise to stripping film preparations.
Another disadvantage is that the film gelatine and, above all, the irregularly distributed silver granules in it, absorb light and thus interfere with, and often render impossible, spectrophotometric evaluation of autoradiographic preparations. Further, the preparation attached to the autoradiogram interferes in the counting of the silver grains in transmitted light; automatic counting can then be carried out only by reflection photometry (Chapter 7).
Photographic reproduction of autoradiograms is comparatively difficult. Silver grains are often masked through the preparation, especially in black and white reproductions. This phenomenon, frequently disagreeably evident in publications, can be circumvented only by special microphotographic techniques; these are described elsewhere (see Sec. 5.2.5.).
Still another shortcoming must be pointed out finally. The stripping technique cannot be employed for autoradiography of water-soluble materials. The method is unsuitable for sections where there is a danger of soluble substances being displaced through remoistening. Attempts

a) b) c) d)

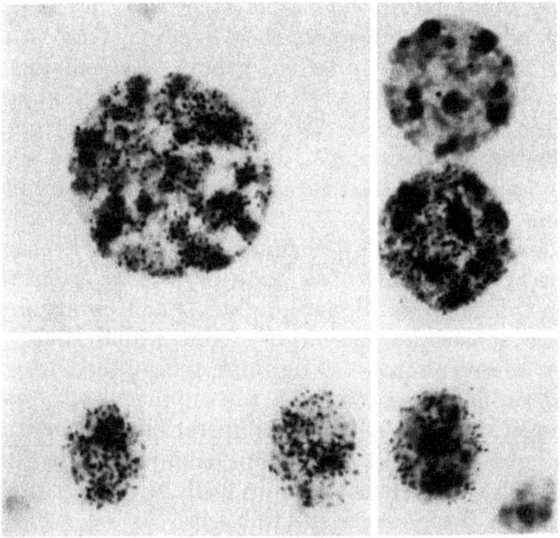

Fig. 48. Comparison of a "pseudo-autoradiogram" resulting from chemography and an autoradiogram induced by tritium β-radiation. From [430]

a) and b) Silver grains chemically induced by orcein prestaining, on the liver cell nuclei of an adult mouse, untreated with radioactive substances; orcein pressing preparation;

c) and d) Typical ^{3}H-thymidine autoradiogram of liver cell nuclei of a 12-day old mouse; pressing preparation, HE-staining after the photographic process. Both magnifications about 1,500 x

have been made to replace by other media (e. g., mercury) the water serving for flotation of the film material, so as to extend the range of application to autoradiography of water-soluble substances. Experiments of this sort have, however, yielded no positive results so far [184]. In another method stripping film was placed on water in the usual way, and then drawn through chloroform followed by further rinsing in anhydrous chloroform and rapid drying in absolute alcohol and air before placing it on to the specimen [74].

5.2.4. Sensitivity and resolution

There are no procedures yet known for determining the sensitivity of photographic emulsions to radiation which can be adapted to autoradiographic practice. The DIN or ASA scales refer to sensitivity towards white light, corresponding to daylight in spectral distribution; they give scarcely any information about sensitivity towards the radiation and energy liberated during radioactive decay processes. It may be roughly taken here also, however, that a larger DIN-value (generally corresponding to larger silver halide grain) is associated with higher sensitivity to radiation. The sensitivity of an emulsion can, however, be varied within certain limits and without change of grain diameter, by adding sensitisers ("dotation"). In this way, special sensitisation or desensitisation can be attained for particular electromagnetic or corpuscular radiation.

It would be ideal if one could determine exactly the average number of energy carriers which have to fall on a crystal in order to convert it into a photographically developable state. Each emulsion would yield a characteristic sensitivity spectrum, from which could be seen immediately how many photons of definite energy lead to exposure of a grain, or what radiation may fall on the emulsion without exposing it. The realisation of this idea encounters obstacles of measuring technique or, at best, demands considerable experimental outlay; one has thus to be content with crude characteristics such as pan- or orthochromatic. Nevertheless, even designations of this sort can be useful in planning autoradiographic investigations. Thus one distinguishes between X-ray film emulsions, specially sensitised for hard or for soft radiation. This distinction is important in the choice of film material for γ-autoradiography since hard and soft emitters occur here. In practice, one is nearly always dependent on experimental testing of the suitability of a film or photoemulsion. Even if film sensitivity spectra of the type mentioned above were available, special tests of autoradiographic suitability would still be necessary. The conversion of the silver halide into a photographically developable condition is significantly influenced by quality and energy distribution of the radiation falling on the film; this is in addition to the actual demands on the resolution, the validity of which can be tested only experimentally. This explains why, even for the most frequently used stripping film, AR 10, only occasional values of sensitivity, resolution and limits of detection are available and which moreover fluctuate considerably, corresponding to the particular experimental conditions [85]. Some data on the so-called grain yield may give information on the sensitivity of stripping films (Table 8). Grain yield is taken as the number of energy carriers, such as α- and β-particles, photons or other quanta and particles, which have to fall on a crystal in order to render it developable photographically. Grain yield is usually determined in practice by relating the absolute number of decay processes in a preparation to the number of silver grains present in the autoradiogram. The existence of spaces between the radiation-sensitive crystals, where radiation is without effect, is not taken into account in this determination method. It must be remembered, moreover, that only half of the radiation is emitted in the direction of the plane of the emulsion and that a part of this is in turn ineffective through being absorbed in the specimen.

The values of MAURER and PRIMBSCH [298] (Table 8) thus deserve special emphasis. They refer to 3 μ sections of methacrylate. The corresponding preparations were ignited and the tritium activity measured in a liquid scintillation counter. Sixteen decay processes per silver grain were found. Only half of the β-particles strikes the emulsion and methacrylate layers of 3 μ thickness possess a self-absorption coefficient for β-radiation of 0.3. For tritium labelling, the real number of electrons leading to

Table 8

Number of decay processes per developable grain of silver in the use of the stripping film *AR 10* (Kodak)

Isotope	Decays/grain	Author(s)
^{3}H	1	HERZ [192]
^{3}H	5 or 20	HUGHES, BOND, BRECHER, CRONKITE, PAINTER, QUASTLER, SHERMAN [211]
^{3}H	20	LAJTHA, OLIVER [246]
^{3}H	10.9	WIMBER, QUASTLER, STEIN, WIMBER [484]
^{3}H	100—200	KISIELESKI, BASERGA, VAUPOTIC [231]
^{3}H	16 or 2.4	MAURER, PRIMBSCH [298]
^{14}C	0.5—0.6	LAJTHA, OLIVER [246]
^{32}P	1.3	HERZ [192]
^{32}P	1.3	LAMERTON, HARRISS [251]
^{32}P	1.3	LAJTHA, OLIVER [246]
^{35}S	0.6	LAMERTON, HARRISS [251]

exposure of a grain emerges thus as 2.4. These factors are not taken into consideration in all the values given in Table 8. Values from different authors cannot therefore be compared. The good agreement for the grain yield for ^{32}P on the one hand and for ^{35}S and ^{14}C on the other may nevertheless be pointed out. Maximum energy, energy distribution and range of the two last-named emitters very nearly agree in each case. It is evident when comparing the values in Table 8 that tritium activity should be less effective than ^{14}C activity. This does not agree with the *energy loss-route relation* (see Chapter 2. and 6.2.1.). An explanation must be sought in either the differing experimental conditions during determination of the grain yields, or a special sensitisation of the emulsion. In this connection we should like to refer to a suggestion of HERZ [194], according to which the sensitivity of stripping films can be enhanced by additives in the developer. This "*hypersensitisation*" has, however, found no widespread use as far as we know.

Information about autoradiographic resolution is even more problematic than comparison of figures for radiation sensitivity, because various things are understood by this term. We consider STEVENS' [426] definition to be the best: resolution is that interval between two radioactively labelled lines of a line grating which can just be detected autoradiographically. We agree with this definition because of its lucidity, even though few experimental values based on it are as yet available. STEVENS [427] and HERZ [193] determined the resolution for ^{131}I to be $2.5u$. It is likely that the resolution for ^{14}C- and ^{3}H-labelled preparations does not differ much from this value, especially since a value of $2.5\,\mu$ was found also for ^{32}P in an analogous way [54; 55]. STEVENS' opinion that the radiation energy is without influence on autoradiographic resolution, provided that the range of the radiation exceeds the thickness of the emulsion layer, appears thus to be confirmed for stripping films.

HERRMANN, HARTMANN and BRUST [189; 190] treated mathematically the relations between radiation energy and resolution.

5.2.5. Microscopy and microphotography of autoradiograms

The mutual relation of preparation and photographic layer undergoes no alteration from the moment when the preparation is covered with stripping film. No particular technical problems of coordination thus arise in the evaluation of stripping film autoradiograms, in contrast to the situation with the contact method. The autoradiograms can be evaluated light-microscopically without more ado. They are covered with a cover glass for inspection at higher magnification, as is customary in light microscopy. Immersion oils may also be used as long as they do not attack the developed photographic layer. The interval between the plane of the preparation and that of the film is, however, unpleasantly noticeable at higher magnifications; only one plane is within the microscopic depth of focus. Yet this effect does not interfere in practice; the possibility of visually separating the two images may even permit a more unprejudiced appraisal. The microscope observer can search out a particular detail of the specimen for more thorough qualitative or quantitative study, based on histological criteria or considerations resulting from the autoradiogram, and he can do this without being consciously influenced by the distribution pattern of the silver grains or by the autoradiographed preparation. This is a considerable advantage.

The autoradiograms can be developed so that large silver grains are formed, expressly for evaluation in transmitted light. Such an autoradiogram practically always shows many background grains; these remain invisible when viewed in transmitted light, yet have a starry sky appearance in dark field lighting.

Over-development, yielding larger grains, naturally does not help with "weak" autoradiograms, i. e., those with only small zones of feeble blackening. One can recommend here only inspection of the silver grain

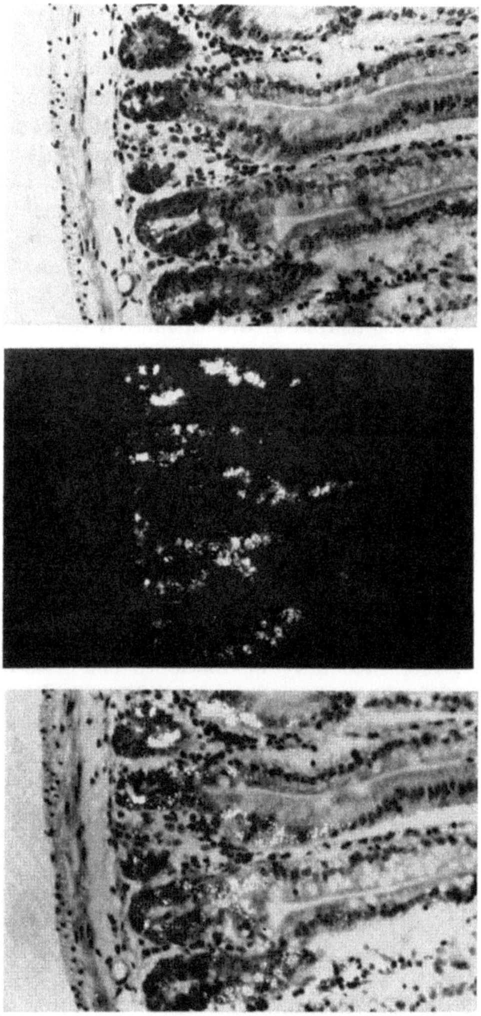

a)

b)

c)

Fig. 49. Some basic ways of microphotographing autoradiograms which are joined with the respective preparation. The preparation is of a stained section of the small intestine of the bushbaby (*Galago demidoffi*). The animal received ^{3}H-thymidine 24 hours before killing. (From [370])

a) Autoradiogram and preparation were photographed together in the bright field of transmitted light. Since silver grains and autoradiographed preparation are in different planes, there is a choice of focussing sharply on either the specimen or the autoradiogram. In both cases the autoradiographic silver grains are masked by the specimen in the background. In the present example, the specimen was focussed;

b) Microphotography of the autoradiogram in incident dark field lighting;

c) Microphotography with combined bright field lighting (transmitted light) and dark field illumination (incident light) (Leitz *Ultropak*, objective 22 x)

distribution in dark field illumination; however, the observer then lacks knowledge of the direct relation of preparation and film.
In microphotography, several possibilities result from the differing planes of preparation and film. As with visual observation, photography in transmitted light requires an optical system directed on to the plane of the object to be photographed. The result is that, in transmitted light, one either records the autoradiogram with good definition above the background of the indistinctly visible preparation; or photographs the preparation with precision and puts up with the fact that the silver grains are scarcely recognisable or are intimated only vaguely. Neither alternative is satisfactory, even less so because the specimen forming the background of the picture always more or less masks the silver grains. A better solution is provided by microphotography of the autoradiogram in dark field illumination, complemented by a second photograph of the appertaining preparation in transmitted light (Fig. 49a & b). Both photographs and the corresponding photographic prints naturally have to be prepared with the same optical magnification in order to preserve the coordination of autoradiographic blackening to specimen details. Useful here is transparent positive paper, on to which the autoradiograms are copied. The copies of autoradiogram and preparation may then simply be laid one on the other to achieve the correct relation to one another. Finally, reference may be made to the possibility of microphotographing autoradiogram and preparation simultaneously. This is accomplished by a combination of incident dark field lighting and bright field illumination in transmitted light. The *Ultropak* system of the firm of Leitz, Wetzlar, W. Germany, is suitable for this purpose [370].
In this Leitz *Ultropak* system, the object is illuminated obliquely from all sides through a ring condenser arranged round the objective. Its illumination aperture is greater than the objective aperture. A vertical illuminator directs the illuminating beam through the objective on to the sample, making use of a half-silvered mirror or asymmetrically placed prisms or a mirror. This last mentioned type of lighting is not really dark field illumination since the illumination aperture has to remain within the framework of the objective aperture. When stripping film autoradiograms are inspected microscopically with the Ultropak equipment, using a weak objective (e. g., the Ultropak objective UO 22 x), the stained section can be studied in transmitted light and the photographic layer in dark field illumination. If both illumination systems are used simultaneously, both pictures can be easily superimposed and, most important, can be microphotographically retained together. In this case, the brightnesses of the two systems are coordinated in order to achieve a picture of section and of emulsion, rich in contrast (Fig. 49c).
Brück has examined the microphotography of unstained autoradiographical preparations [66].

5.3. Autoradiography with "liquid" emulsions

BÉLANGER and LEBLOND [34; 40] describe a technique in which a liquid emulsion is thinly painted on to the preparation under investigation. This method assures the most intimate contact between specimen and radiation-sensitive layer. Moreover, an optimum layer thickness can be obtained by using suitably diluted emulsions. These expectations have been largely realised.

Table 9

Data on some emulsions employed for liquid emulsion technique; sensitivities to radiation on the Ilford scale. According to A. W. ROGERS (Section 9.2., VIII)

Manufacturer	Crystal diameter (μ)	Sensitivity 0	1	2	3	4	5
Ilford	0.27	G0	G1	G2	G3	G4	G5
Ilford	0.20	K0	K1	K2	K3	K4	K5
Ilford	0.15	L0	L1	L2	L3	L4	
Eastman-Kodak	0.40						NTB-4
Eastman-Kodak	0.30		NTA	NTB	NTB-2		NTB-3
Eastman-Kodak	0.04			NTE			
Agfa-Gevaert	0.15						NUC 7.15
Agfa-Gevaert	0.07				NUC 3.07		

The nuclear track emulsions developed for nuclear physics interests are especially suitable for this technique and for the dipping technique described later. Table 9 gives some information about them.

Emulsions quoted in column 0 (Table 9) are suitable only for α-autoradiography. They do not record β-particles. The emulsions in the following columns are suitable for detecting lower energy β-emitters and therefore especially tritium and ^{125}I. Radiocarbon and ^{35}S of approximately equal energy are detected by emulsions in columns 4 and 5. Those completely on the right-hand side of the table may be used for β-track autoradiography (Sec. 7.2.).

The emulsions are available commercially in colloidal state as gels. They should be stored and treated in accordance with the directions of the manufacturers. The most suitable temperature at which they remain usable for a longer period is about +4° C. It appears that irreversible changes take place in the gelatine at lower temperatures; this makes the gelatine unusable. The emulsions can be kept for only a limited time, given mostly by the manufacturers as about 2 months. One should naturally employ the dark room lighting prescribed for work with the particular liquid emulsion. The recommended air humidity should also be respected since emulsion layers which have dried out too much often have increased background.

For use in autoradiographic work the emulsions are first liquefied by warming in a water bath. The temperature — including that of the water bath! — should not exceed 40—45° C. The emulsions should generally be diluted with distilled water before further use. The extent of dilution is governed by the nature of the emitter to be detected and the subsequent evaluation of the autoradiogram. To attain the highest possible resolution, the thickness of the emulsion ought to be from 1 to 2 μ after application and evaporation of the water. Still thicker layers should be used for quantitative evaluations. Bélanger and Leblond spread the emulsion over the preparation with a fine brush. They used a pre-warmed pipette for dropping a small amount of emulsion on the likewise pre-warmed specimen surface. The preparations thus made are maintained at 40° C for about 1 minute so that the emulsion can run uniformly after spreading. The preparation is finally left to cool in a horizontal position and the emulsion then gelatinises and dries firmly. Non-uniform emulsions may be formed in this procedure, resulting in inhomogeneities in thickness and distribution of silver crystals in the film layer. These undesirable effects can be avoided through use of a modified technique, frequently used. The slides carrying the specimens are dipped into the warmed, diluted emulsion until the preparation is completely covered with emulsion. The slides are slowly withdrawn from the solution and then, by holding them vertically, the emulsion runs into a thin layer which is relatively homogeneous and which adheres well. This procedure is termed *dipping* technique [215; 216; 217; 240; 305]. The dilution of the emulsion needed to prepare the desired layer thickness must be ascertained in preliminary experiments with appropriate dilution series. It is between 1 and 10 parts of water per part (volume) of emulsion (cf Table 11).

The preparations are exposed at ca +4° C in light-tight preparation boxes. In publications so far, no consistent opinion has been advanced whether the presence of a drying agent has any influence on background value or fading of the latent image or has any chemographic effect. This applies also to the composition of the atmosphere in which the preparations are to be exposed [194].

The techniques described here, in which aqueous emulsions are brought into contact with the preparations, are restricted to detection of those substances which are bound to macromolecular structures and hence have low water solubility. Many experiments have been undertaken to extend the range of application by using suitable protective layers to prevent the penetration of moisture into the preparations. A layer of celloidin is recommended, prepared by repeated immersion in a 1% solution of celloidin in a mixture of ether and alcohol. Protective layers of PVC (polyvinyl chloride) are used also. These are obtained either by placing a drop of 6.4% PVC solution on water and passing the slide under the film, or laying the section on the film; or by immersing the slide in dilute PVC solutions. The average thickness of such protective films is 0.12—0.24 μ. The disadvantages of intermediate layers of this sort are widely known: both the resolution in tritium autoradiography and the ability to stain the preparations are affected [394].

Liquid emulsion technique, like stripping technique, is inapplicable to studies of water-soluble substances. Since the former has not even the advantage of reproducible layer thickness and quality, it has been pushed more and more into the background in recent years by the stripping technique. Both methods are susceptible to the difficulties associated with the staining of histological preparations.

The are two possibilities for staining: it is done either before the emulsion is applied or after photographic development. Many risks threaten the autoradiography of preparations which have already been stained. These are due to interaction of the dye with the silver halide of the photographic layer. The positive chemographic action of some dyes is known.

Positive chemography through dyes has already been encountered in connection with the stripping technique (Fig. 48). By *negative chemography* is understood the phenomenon of insufficient blackening of certain parts of an autoradiogram despite adequate activity and exposure time; it is evidently due to oxidation of the latent autoradiographic image.

THURSTON and JOFTES [441] assessed relatively frequently used staining methods from the point of view of possible sources of error in autoradiographic technique. Dyes which may be employed before application of the emulsion without fear of artefacts include: Feulgen Fast Green, haematoxylin-phloxine and aldehyde-fuchsin-PAS (periodate Schiff). The best results in staining after photographic development were obtained with: Celestine Blue, Mayer's haemalum, Metanil Yellow-iron-haematoxylin, lithium carmine-picric acid, Weigert's acid iron-haematoxylin, methyl green-pyronine, indigo carmine-picric acid and toluidine blue. The gelatine layer is scarcely coloured. Amongst the most suitable dyes for staining before coating with emulsion and again after photographic development and fixing are: trichrome-PAS, haematoxylin-eosin and aniline blue-carbolfuchsin. One must always check of course whether displacement or decrease of radioactivity occurs in the histological preparation as a result of washing out the labelled substance. VON DEIMLING, WITSCH and ROSSNER [93] studied methods of PAS and Feulgen staining of developed autoradiographed paraffin sections.

5.4. Methods for autoradiography of displaceable substances

5.4.1. Preliminary remarks

The methods treated in the preceding sections fail when the substances to be detected are easily soluble in the solvents or fixation media commonly used for histological preparations. The action merely of atmospheric moisture or of water from the photographic emulsion can bring about undesirable displacements of the labelled compounds or even dissolve them out.

That conventional autoradiographic techniques are restricted to the virtually insoluble, especially covalent compounds, has long been known. The extent to which one has to reckon with displacements is less well known. BLANCK and co-workers [52] report that nearly 40% of phosphorus-containing cell constituents, which can be labelled with ^{32}P are extracted with formalin or Bouin solution. The substances extracted include the large number of simply phosphorylated compounds and nucleic acid precursors and also short nucleotide chains, probably up to a molecular weight of 2,000 or more. VINCENT [458] reports that ribonucleic acid (RNA) also can be extracted during usual fixation of starfish oocyte nucleoli. SCHNEIDER and MAURER [399] review the possible loss of RNA and its precursors from various mouse tissues after tagging with ^{3}H-cytidine. KOPRIWA and LEBLOND [240] report similar results on mouse liver. Loss of material occurs also during fixation of human brain tissue with formalin [400]. The examples show that, for preparing autoradiograms of biological specimens, the fixation process must be chosen carefully or, best of all, chemical fixation with solvents should be renounced.

FEINENDEGEN [130] and APPLETON [13] have compiled reviews of the attempts at autoradiographical depiction of water-soluble substances.

The consistent elimination of all those influences which might clearly change the original distribution and allocation of the radioactivity during preparation of histological specimens and their autoradiograms means that practically only combinations of the freeze-drying or freeze section technique with the contact autoradiographic procedure satisfy the requirements for avoiding displacements. To attain maximum resolution, especially in work with ^{3}H-labelled substances, it is desirable to establish direct contact between specimen and photoemulsion without any adhering intermediate layer. Such layers would moreover only create further doubt concerning their action on the substance distribution in the preparation.

Micro-histoautoradiography of diffusible substances is accomplished chiefly at the present time according to APPLETON's procedure [10—13], a type of inversion method [33]; or according to the contact method based on the early technique of FITZGERALD and co-workers [138] now further adapted for use with diffusible labelled substances by WERNER and co-workers [473—481; 60] and by STUMPF and ROTH [433; 434].

5.4.2. APPLETON's method

The tissue samples are first frozen in isopentane, cooled in liquid nitrogen and kept some time in liquid nitrogen. Frozen sections of 4—6 μ thickness are then prepared in a cryostat at —30° C. These are transferred in safety light (*Kodak Wratten Series 1*) to pre-cooled slides at —5° C (Fig. 50). The slides have been previously coated with stripping film so that the emulsion layer is on the outside. Under the conditions used, the histological section adheres to the photographic layer without melting. The reason for this adhesion is still disputed. The preparations, which have not thawed at any point, are exposed at —25° C. Fixation is carried out at room temperature in alcohol containing 5% acetic acid and this is followed by washing, developing and staining. Finally, the preparation + adhering film is transferred to a glass slide so that the section lies between the glass and the emulsion (Fig. 50).
Compared to the contact method described below, APPLETON's method seems complicated to us and especially poorly suited to routine application with large series of sections. It is doubtful whether the basic idea of consistently handling deep-frozen material really ensures that no displacements occur through diffusion or convection. Probably it is the cutting process rather than the conditions of exposure which are responsible for changes taking place in the substance distribution (cf Section 4.3.2.); this would then be the absolutely deciding factor in the autoradiography of easily displaceable materials. The relatively simple evaluation of the preparations may be regarded as an advantage over the contact method which demands a greater technical outlay. APPLETON's method gets cleverly round the difficulties of the normal stripping procedure by using a reversal technique [33]; it shares with the stripping procedure, however, those disadvantages which can arise during the photographic process through the contact of emulsion and preparation (see Section 5.3.).

5.4.3. Contact autoradiography

The degree of coordination of film blackening with source of radiation in the specimen which can be attained in the autoradiographic contact method is less than that in procedures which are based on virtually indissoluble contact between film layer and specimen. Nevertheless, contact autoradiography is of great practical significance because it

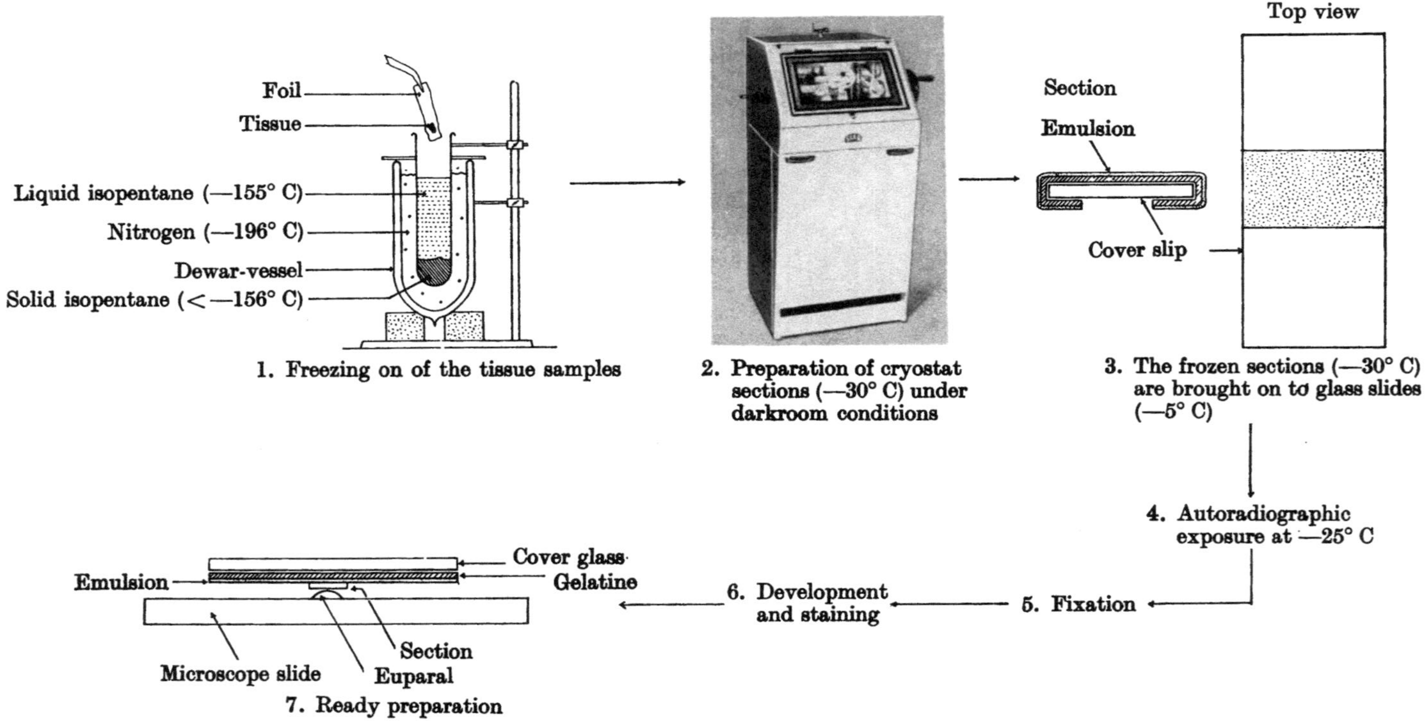

Fig. 50. Scheme of APPLETON's method [13]. Details in text

permits detection of *all* labelled substances — hence also dissolved or easily diffusible — which are not noticeably volatile. The procedures of Werner and co-workers, described below and especially worked out with this in mind, are suitable in conjunction with the histological frozen section technique and also for preparations made according to the freeze drying technique [60; 473—481]. They have been often taken over and modified [150].

5.4.3.1. Frozen sections

The specimens are frozen on freeze blocks by means of solid carbon dioxide and then kept for several hours in a sealed polyethylene bag, intended to protect from moisture (see Section 4.3.2.) in a cryostat at —25° C. Sections of ca 10 μ thickness are prepared and brought on to cooled slides stored in the cryostat. The frozen sections are stretched and fixed by pressing a finger against the slide from underneath to warm it temporarily to a few degrees above zero.
Surprisingly, scarcely any detectable displacements are caused through this brief "thawing" of the sections. This is possibly explained by the fact that the cell walls suffer sensibly no mechanical damage through freezing. One may, however, expect smudges during application of the frozen section technique when the labelled substance is extra-cellular, e. g., in the intestinal lumen or collecting tubes of the kidneys. These are probably partly caused by the cutting procedure since brief melting of the preparation in the immediate neighbourhood of the knife edge naturally cannot be avoided (cf Section 4.3.2.). After thawing, the sections lie flat on the slide and stick adequately. The low atmospheric humidity in the cryostat must not increase very much during cutting. This can be accomplished by sealing the arm inlets of the cryostat with foam rubber padding during use. Before the sections are removed they should be freeze dried by keeping open for several hours in the cryostat. The glass slide must be previously warmed to about room temperature (within the cryostat) with a finger or small hot plate, so that no water condenses on the tissue section when it is taken out.

5.4.3.2. Paraffin sections

The procedure in the freeze drying method is as follows: The organ samples are taken as quickly as possible from the killed animal. Small parts of them are cooled to about —160° C in isopentane which is viscous at this temperature. Fast work is necessary so that there is negligible postmortal change in the distribution of the substances to be detected. Uncertainty still reigns about the extent to which postmortal enzymatic and diffusion processes occur; they vary anyhow from substance to substance [286]. The frozen organ parts are transferred to glass tubes, precooled to —30° to —40° C. These contain paraffin wax which has been degassed in vacuo. They are left 3 to 4 days here under a constant low pressure of 10^{-3} mm mercury. On the last day, the temperature of the bath is gradually raised from —30° C to room temperature. The wax in the tube is then melted by dipping the tube into a water bath. The dried pieces of organ sink into the paraffin wax and are left there at +65° C for a further half-hour. They are then poured out and worked into paraffin wax sections. These are placed on slides which have been prepared with egg-white-glycerol and are cautiously pressed down with, for example, a teflon plate or piece of blotting paper. The sections are left on the extension table for a while at +37° C and are then either brought into contact with the photo-emulsion without any further pre-treatment, or are first deparaffined with absolutely anhydrous xylene. Covering with the photographic layer immediately after deparaffining the sections is recommended in order to avoid uptake of atmospheric moisture.

5.4.3.3. Film material, exposure and development

The *G 5* Ilford emulsion has proved highly satisfactory film material. It is available in gel form. This is diluted 1 : 1 with distilled water and warmed to 40—42° C. For preparing the film material, strips of 2 × ca 20 cm are cut from an optically isotropic film base, coated with adhesive. It is procured as X-ray film sheet. Using *Tesafilm D* (similar to *Scotch tape*), these strips are stuck firmly along their edges to a plastic plate, previously warmed to about 40° C. A drop of the warmed emulsion is then placed on the areas between the Tesafilm strips on the film base and is immediately spread out uniformly along the length, using the rounded narrow edge of a slide. After the emulsion has dried, the *Tesafilm* is removed and pieces of about 2 × 2 cm are cut out of the resulting film strip. Any non-uniformly covered pieces are discarded. The film base must not be touched with the bare fingers during this procedure [481].
The emulsion-coated film plates are laid against the organ section (coated side towards it), covered with a second slide which is about 4 cm shorter and then the bundle is pressed together with a clamp. The purpose of the second slide is to exert a uniform pressure on the self-prepared flexible pieces of film (Fig. 51). The procedure is considerably easier when one starts with slides already coated with the same film layer; these are commercially available.
One can easily prepare coated slides oneself also by dipping. The emulsion must adhere sufficiently firmly to the glass. In our experience, this is accomplished satisfactorily by adding the surface-active material *Hostapon T* (Farbwerke Hoechst AG, W. Germany). We add 5 drops of a 10% Hostapon solution to 25 ml water, then making up the total volume to 50 ml with Ilford *G 5* emulsion; during this, the vessel is maintained at 40—42° C in a water bath. After mixing (avoid foaming!),

the temperature is kept at 30° C and a carefully cleaned slide dipped into the emulsion. The slide is then withdrawn with as smooth a movement as possible, excess emulsion is wiped from the edge and the slide, now coated on both sides, is placed in a sloping position in the grooves of a home-made shelf. After about 12 hours, these coated slides can be used for covering histological sections in the same way as described in connection with the emulsion-coated sheet. One should

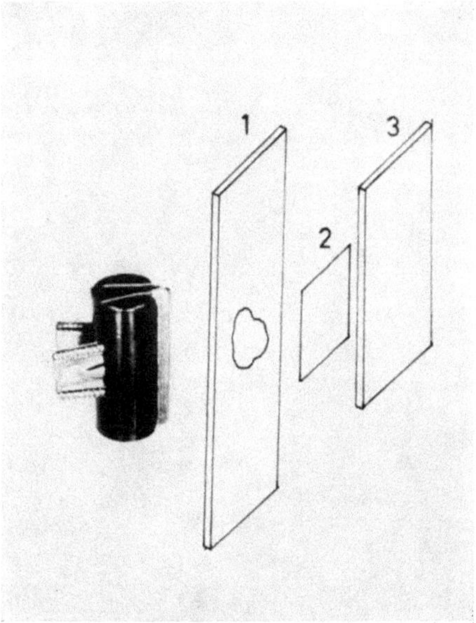

Fig. 51. Components and arrangement for autoradiographic exposure. 1 — Slide with organ section; 2 — sheet with photo-emulsion; 3 — small slide; 4 — clamp for pressing together the whole arrangement. From [481]

take care that the emulsion coating is homogeneous where it is placed against the section. The side of the emulsion facing the section can be marked with a pencil.

The preparations are stored in the usual preparation boxes, with small linen bags containing silica gel as drying agent. The boxes are enveloped in light-tight plastic bags and kept in a refrigerator at +4° C. After autoradiographic exposure, the preparation boxes are removed from the refrigerator and left some hours at room temperature. This prevents condensation of water on the film or section when the boxes are opened. Histological preparations can be stained in the usual way after autoradiography.

It is most convenient to employ the slide holders generally used in histological staining technique in photographic development of emulsion-

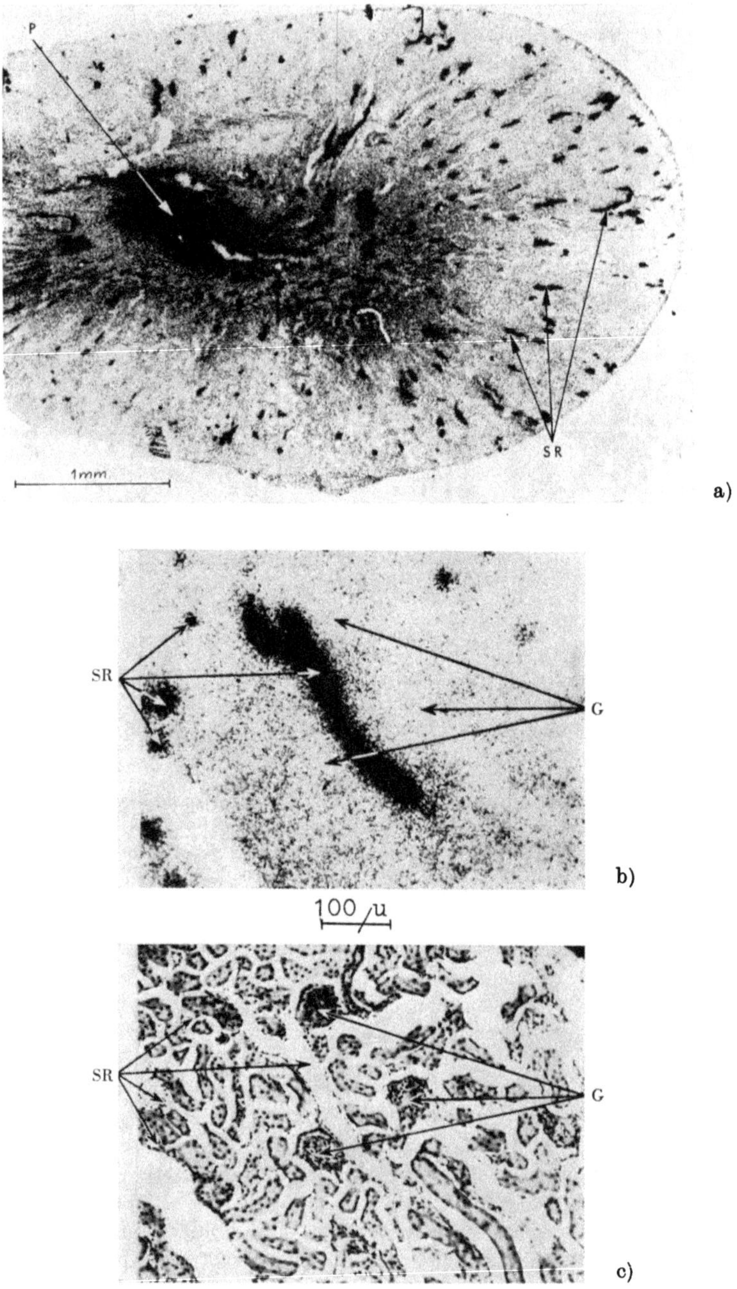
P
SR
1mm
a)
SR
G
b)
100 μ
SR
G
c)

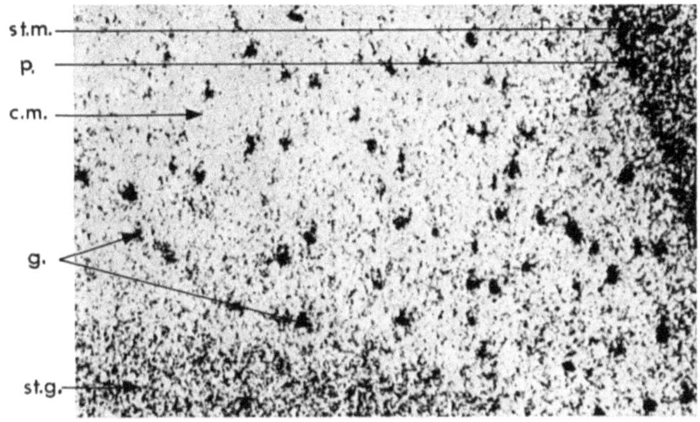

d)

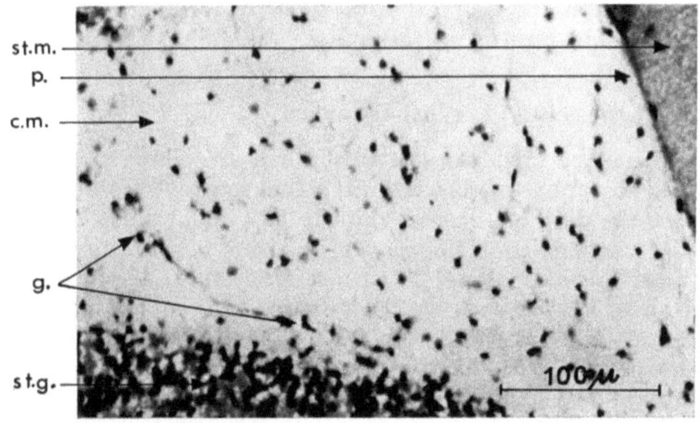

e)

Figs. 52 d and e. Autoradiogram (d) and frozen section (e) from the cerebellum of a rat. 54 μl = 180 μC of ^{3}H-glutamic acid, dissolved in physiological NaCl, were injected into the left lateral ventricle by means of a calibrated glass sphere, 95 min before killing. Before exposure, the section was freed from surface cholesterol crystals by sprinkling with xylene; the xylene was immediately sucked off. MAY-GRÜNWALD-GIEMSA staining after autoradiographic exposure. 12 weeks exposure

st. m. = *stratum moleculare*, p = *pia*, c. m. = *corpus medullare*, g = *glia*, st. g. = *stratum granulosum*

← Figs. 52 a—c

a) Contact autoradiogram of the kidney section of a mouse, prepared according to the freeze drying technique, after i. p. injection of an aqueous solution of polytopic labelled ^{3}H-atropine sulphate. Killed 10 min after injection. 5 weeks exposure. Preparation about 5 mm long;

b) Section of a);

c) Section of the histological preparation corresponding to b), after HE-staining

Figs. 52 b and c from [481]

G = glomerulus, P = papillae, SR = collecting tube

coated slides. The self-prepared film pieces are hung in steel frames, specially employed for development of X-ray dental films [481]. Following 6 min development in *D 19b* (Kodak) at 20° C, the film is briefly rinsed in tap water, fixed and again washed in running tap water. The emulsion-coated pieces of film must be left in distilled water for a further hour after this. In contrast, rinsing with distilled water must be brief with both the ready-made and the self-prepared emulsion-coated slides. Subsequent drying must be in dust-free air.
The reverse side of the self-prepared emulsion-coated slides, which shows no autoradiographic blackening, is wiped clean during the washing after fixing. Any residues still remaining can be finally removed with aqueous ammonia solution after drying. The autoradiogram is embedded with a cover glass in *Eukitt* and the caption preserved with Zaponlack. The pieces of film are fastened with *Eukitt* to ordinary glass slides so that the autoradiogram is on the inside.

5.4.3.4. Artefacts caused by crystal depositions

Reference must be made to artefacts which are observed especially in the autoradiography of brain and spinal marrow frozen sections*. Crystals can be detected on the white matter about a day after storage of cryostat sections for some hours at room temperature (Fig. 53a). They are crystals of cholesterol and can occasionally be recognised with the naked eye. They absorb the ^{3}H-radiation of the layer beneath them, so that no more activity can be recognised autoradiographically on the sites concerned (Figs 53b and c). Artefacts of this sort can be avoided

* Korr, H., H. A. Fischer, N. Seiler and G. Werner: Cholesterinkristalle in Kryostat-Gefrierschnitten von nervösem Gewebe als Ursache von Artefakten in Autoradiogrammen. Histochemie **23** (1970) 138.

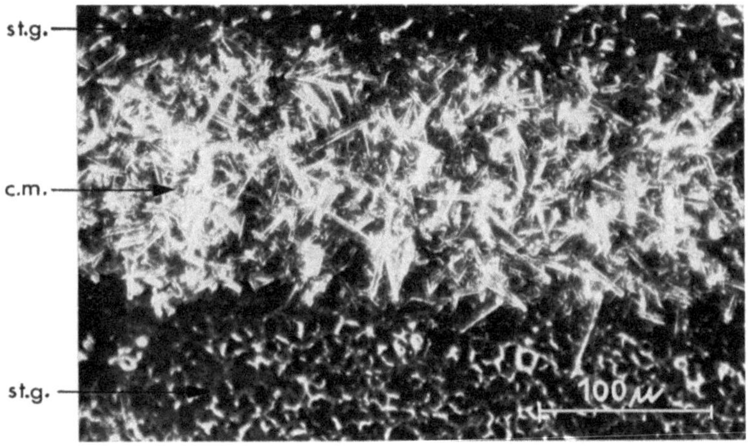

a)

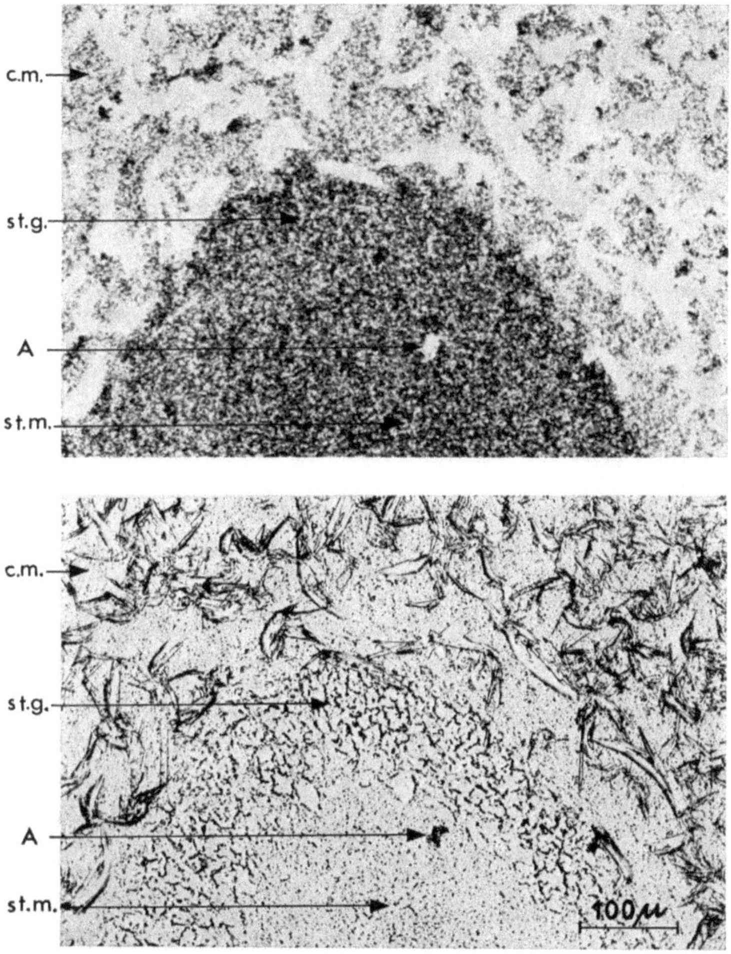

b)

c)

Fig. 53. Artefacts on contact autoradiograms of frozen sections, caused by crystal formation

a) Cholesterol crystals on unstained section of the cerebellum of a *Hapale jacchus*. Dark field photograph;

b) and c) Autoradiogram and unstained section from the same region in bright field illumination. The artefacts in the autoradiogram, due to crystals on the section, are clearly recognisable (cf Section 5.4.3.4.)

Preparation: *Hapale jacchus*, 8 hours after dosage of 64 mC ^{3}H-*encephabol* (Merck, Darmstadt, W. Germany) (i. p. and per os)

st. g. = *stratum granulosum*, c. m. = *corpus medullare*, st. m. = *stratum moleculare*, A = artefact, e. g., through contamination with foreign body

only by preventing crystal formation. Crystals are not observed as long as frozen sections are continuously subjected to temperatures below —20° C. Even brief warming to ambient temperature initiates crystal formation. Artefacts may be circumvented by consistent work at suitably low temperature; this includes also the coating with photo-emulsion and autoradiographic exposure. This would mean practically resorting to APPLETON's procedure [13]. We consider that routine work with a large number of sections is no longer possible under these conditions and have worked out the procedure described below* in order to prevent appearance of crystalline cholesterol on frozen sections.
The sections prepared in the cryostat (see Sec. 5.4.3.1.) are transferred to a closed vessel (Petri dish) at +80° C immediately after removal from the cryostat; the vessel contains dry paraformaldehyde (trioxymethylene). Ca 12 hours treatment with the formaldehyde atmosphere thus yielded hinders all subsequent formation of crystals on the dry sections.

5.4.4. Advantages and disadvantages of the contact method

The principal advantage of the contact procedure is that it is suitable for all labelled substances in biological material, provided that they are not too volatile under the given experimental conditions. Further, the procedure is relatively easy to carry out; this allows routine autoradiography at acceptable speed of continously delivered serial sections. As many contact autoradiograms as desired can be prepared from one and the same preparation. This is important with preparations of highly varied activity distribution, where the best evaluation demands a varied choice of exposure time. Direct histochemical studies of the autoradiographed specimen are possible also, since film and section are separated after autoradiographic exposure. Unlike in other procedures, one is therefore not dependent on reference investigations on neighbouring sections. Eliminated also, of course, are those interfering influences associated with the stripping procedure, for example, through having to treat film and preparation together with the reagents for photographic development. Chemographic effects resulting from this in other procedures do not arise in the contact procedure. Moreover, the emulsion cannot interfere with the staining reactions.
A disadvantage is the necessarily more difficult evaluation of the autoradiograms, since there is no longer direct contact between film and preparation. Autoradiographic blackening and specimen detail can therefore be coordinated only when there is the possibility of bringing autoradiogram and histological preparation together again in their original congruence. The solution of this problem of coordination (Chapter 5.4.5.) was critical for the routine application of the contact method to auto-

---

* See footnote p. 86.

radiography of microscopic specimens. The autoradiogram can be observed independently of the specimen and this offers a final advantage of quantitative evaluation through procedures of light absorption; there is no adhering preparation which absorbs light and influences the measurement [135] (Section 7.3.).

5.4.5. Topographic localisation of silver grains in contact autoradiography

Various ways have been attempted from time to time of bringing tissue and film again into coincidence after staining the histological preparation or following development of the autoradiogram. They can then be inspected and evaluated together. For example, crosses have been drawn on the slide with radioactive ink before exposure. These were registered in the photographic emulsion and served as marks to reestablish more easily the congruence of section and autoradiogram [202]. Hoecker and Roofe [198] utilised a folding apparatus, in which the sections were situated on a flexible slide support. After autoradiographic exposure, emulsion and section could be folded away from each other and be treated (developed and stained) separately.
Other authors have localised tracks of α-particles in contact autoradiograms by photographing as prints the previously stained tissue sections after exposure; this was done on the same emulsion, on which the tracks were already present as latent images. The tissue then appears as a sort of silhouette on which the autoradiogram is superimposed. This procedure is of course limited to α-particle tracks since the blackening yielded by β-particles cannot be distinguished from that due to visible light [397; 396].
All these procedures have the disadvantage that routine work is difficult or limited to one particular type of radiation. Progress came with the development of an apparatus allowing preparation and associated contact autoradiogram to be focussed microscopically in the same optical plane (Fig. 54). Two identical microscopes are fixed to a mutual base. One of them possesses its own illumination system. Autoradiogram and histological preparation are attached to two swivel tables and can be moved, independently of each other, in two coordinate directions. One microscope is equipped with a binocular. By means of an optical system, consisting of two prisms and lateral tubes, the image of the object in the second microscope can be projected into the optical path of the first. In this way, both preparations can be focussed in the same optical plane. Two identical preparations can be focussed congruently, provided that the optical conditions are the same in both image planes. This equipment therefore fulfils all requirements for correct coordination of autoradiogram and histological preparation. A microscope stage of adjustable height permits compensation of any differences in the thickness of the slide used. It may also be mentioned that the stages of

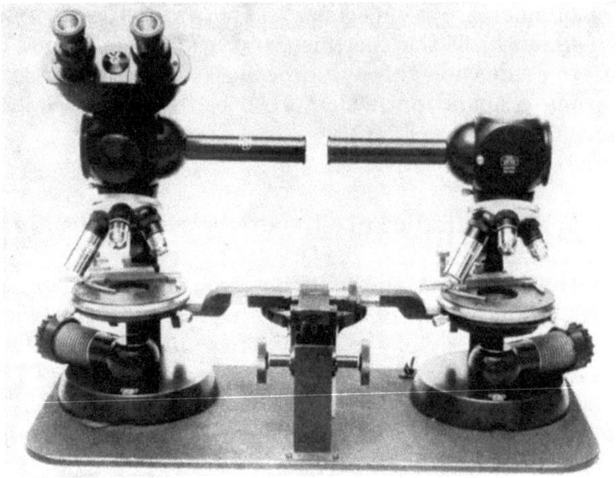

Fig. 54. Double microscope equipment for coordinating autoradiographic blackening on histological structures in the contact autoradiography of light microscopic preparations, according to WERNER et al [137]. See text for explanation

both microscopes can be transported simultaneously horizontally or vertically. If the specimens are rightly orientated, every detail can be observed without losing the existing optical superimposition. This method provides the desired exact congruence of autoradiogram and section without much effort by either first optically superimposing their exterior contours at low magnification; or bringing other already known, strikingly evident details of the specimen into coincidence with their corresponding feature in the autoradiogram. If only one of the two preparations is to be inspected, the image of the complementary object may be stopped down by reducing the intensity of its illumination.

This double microscope has proved most useful in the topographical evaluation of our autoradiograms.

Similar apparatus is now also commercially available. The firm of Leitz, for example, combines two *Ortholux* microscopes with a so-called Vergleichsbrücke which also permits two identical preparations to be optically superimposed. Unfortunately, simultaneous transport of preparations is not possible with this instrument. Preparations to be compared thus always have to be newly adjusted to each other with every fresh microscope position. Rapid scrutiny of autoradiograms, especially necessary in routine studies, is thus made much more difficult and is impeded, at least at high magnifications.

6. AUTORADIOGRAPHY OF ELECTRON-MICROSCOPE SPECIMENS

6.1. Introduction

The resolution of light-microscopic autoradiography (Chapter 5.) attains about 2 to 3 μ in favourable cases; this just enables crude allocations to be made in the intracellular domain. Knowledge of cell structure has been considerably extended through the application of electron microscopy; yet the state of development of high resolution autoradiography is not regarded as adequate with regard to cytochemical problems.

The initial impulses towards development of such autoradiographic techniques, reconcilable with the technical features of electron microscopy, go back to HAMM and COMER [178] and LIQUIER-MILWARD [271]. Since then, a larger number of publications on techniques of electron microscopic autoradiography has come out. In our opinion, the methodological aspect cannot, however, be regarded as settled or mature.

In the present chapter, we intend to describe the most important contributions hitherto made to electron-microscopic autoradiographic technique and to adopt a critical attitude to the methods. So far there have been over 300 publications with special reference to electron-microscope autoradiography; we must therefore limit ourselves here to a few examples only*. Theoretical considerations are dealt with only briefly in order to be able to present the problems of method, slanted particularly for practical application.

The question of the theoretically attainable resolution will be treated first, since the combination of autoradiography and electron microscopy involves some special features of methodological nature. This applies in particular to the coordination of the silver grains to autoradiographed specimen. As will be illustrated in individual cases, the cardinal problem is the differing resolution of autoradiogram and electron microscope picture. The best autoradiographic resolution so far attained is about 100 times inferior to that of the electron microscope. The situation is thus in complete contrast to that in light microscope autoradiography [426; 427].

---

* Reviews see p. 191; see also D. NEUMANN [320].

6.2. Resolution

6.2.1. Theoretical considerations

The first fundamental contribution towards a mathematical grasp of the factors governing resolution is by DONIACH and PELC [108]. Their considerations were based on an ideal point source of light. HERRMANN, HARTMANN and BRUST [189] undertook a mathematically soundly based calculation of the relation between resolution and maximum energy of an emitter; they bore in mind the fact that labelled specimens in autoradiography have finite size. Unfortunately both these studies were based on stripping emulsions of about 3 μ thickness. Their basic models and conceptions cannot thus be directly applied for information in electron-microscope autoradiography. Further points are:

1. Extremely thin photographic layers with a high content of silver halide are used in electron-microscope autoradiography, in contrast to other applications; in the ideal case, the layer would consist of a single layer of halide grain. The physico-chemical properties of such thin radiation-sensitive layers differ markedly from those of thicker film material.

2. Apart from the differing nature and structure of the photographic emulsion, DONIACH and PELC's model is valid only for thicker layers. Just as different darkening properties are associated with thinner film layers, so one must take into consideration radiation effects with the unavoidably very thin electron-microscopic preparations which would be negligible with thicker preparations. The route taken by an emitted low-energy β-particle through ionisable material is characterised by frequent elastic and inelastic collisions; these bring about a continued change of direction of particle path. This change must be considered in a theoretical treatment of resolution. In no case is it permissible in those dimensions attainable in electron-microscopic magnification to imagine the radiation emitting linearly in all directions from a point source; only low-energy emitters (see Section 6.8.) may be used and scattering is relatively strong.

Despite these difficulties, the resolution of electron-microscope autoradiograms has been the object of various mathematical treatments [77; 346; 22] in which the peculiarities just mentioned have been considered in part. CARO [77] quoted optimistically about 860 Å as the maximum attainable resolution for tritium-containing preparations. He considered a specimen in which a point radiation source is situated 500 Å beneath a photographic emulsion with silver halide of average grain diameter of 1,000 Å (Fig. 55). He took the densities of the specimen to be autoradiographed and of the gelatine component of the radiation-sensitive emulsion to be 1.1. LEA* had already estimated the range

* LEA, D. E.: "Actions of Radiations on Living Cells," Cambridge Univ. Press, London 1956.

spectrum for a medium of unit density, based on the known energy and range spectrum of the radiation emitted from tritium in vacuo. CARO extrapolated these data for media of density 1.1 and found that 20% of the radiation impinges on the emulsion when the point source and emulsion are 1 μ apart. If this is increased to 2 μ, the amount of incident radiation rises by only a further 2%. In other words, increasing the thickness of the section to more than 2 μ should have no further influence on the time of exposure and resolution. As far as we know, this result, of interest for autoradiography of microscopic preparations, has not so far been tested experimentally.

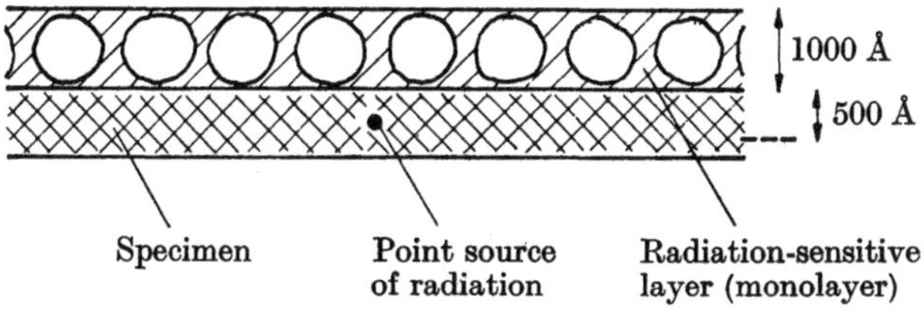

Fig. 55. Scheme on which CARO's estimate of maximum resolution is based. Details in the text

CARO next investigated the distribution of radiation around two sources of radiation of identical intensity, as a function of their separation (Fig. 56). He utilised the radiation distribution around a single point source, relatively easily expressed quantitatively. He thus determined the separation at which both emitting sources could still be separately distinguished with certainty, as seen through darkening of the photographic layer. RAYLEIGH's postulate was taken as the criterion of "still resolvable"; according to this, resolution is possible when the intensity of the radiation superposed on the line joining the points of origin

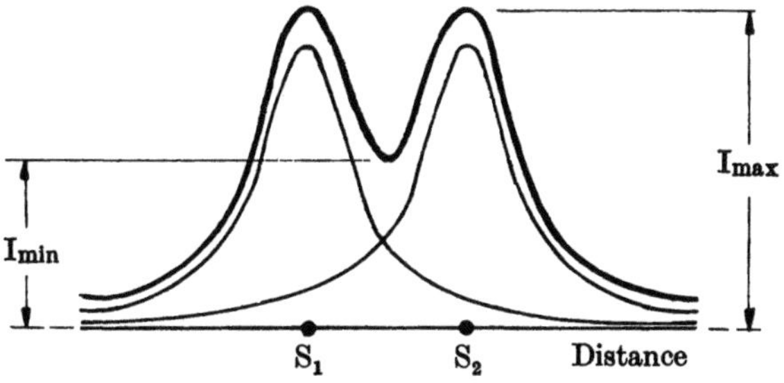

Fig. 56. Distribution of radiation around two point radiation sources S_1 and S_2. RAYLEIGH's criterion requires $I_{min} \geqq \frac{I_{max}}{2}$ to be able to distinguish the two sources

differs from the maximum intensity by at least 50% (Fig. 56). CARO found, as already mentioned, that an interval of 860 Å can still be resolved. This means that the resolution corresponds approximately to the diameter of the silver halide crystals in the emulsion. CARO was able to confirm experimentally the order of magnitude determined by him for the resolution. Other authors have had similar results [346; 22].

6.2.2. Attainable resolution

Theoretical estimates of the type dealt with above have certainly shared in stimulating the numerous experimental efforts to develop generally practicable methods. Nevertheless, the techniques which have been hitherto proposed have not fulfilled the hopes placed in them. The discrepancy between the theoretically possible and the practically attainable resolutions may be explained in our opinion by the fact that certain factors have been inadequately taken into consideration in the theoretical treatment. These factors are:

1. the fact that the photographic layer may no longer be regarded as a homogeneous layer,
2. the photographic process,
3. the process of delivery or transfer of radiation energy to the photographic emulsion,
4. the magnitude of the time of exposure and the background.

Concerning 1: Every photographic emulsion consists of at least two components of differing mechanical density. These are the silver halide crystals (density 6.47) as the radiation-sensitive component, and a binder, gelatine (density ca 1.1). Emulsions of high silver halide content and smallest possible crystal diameter, yielding a homogeneous and compact covering of the surface of the preparation, must be used in electron-microscope autoradiography. The grain diameter of fine-grain emulsions, the preparation of which in greater amounts has become only recently technically possible, is about 700—1000 Å. It is thus of the order of magnitude of the theoretically realisable resolution.
The considerations which led to the theoretical value of 860 Å for the resolution included the RAYLEIGH criterion. Subsequently it was tacitly assumed, however, that a radiation intensity, reduced to a half, necessarily yields a correspondingly diminished blackening intensity on the film. This is possible only with film material, which, in these dimensions (the region of 1000 Å), can reproduce differences in blackening intensity proportional to the radiation. This cannot be accomplished, however, with the 500—1000 Å grains of present-day emulsions!

Concerning 2: The misgivings about the theoretical judgment of resolution which result from still incomplete knowledge of the photographic processes are fourfold:

a) there is no proof that the autoradiographic silver grains are formed exactly in those regions where the latent image nucleates are created. One is even inclined to believe nowadays that the latent image does not necessarily have to be at that spot on the crystal which is struck by the electron or photon*;

b) during photographic development, a silver nucleate grows probably from the region of the latent image, depending on the developing conditions. This nucleate takes the form of a worm-like filament which repeatedly meanders and may even grow almost linearly from its place of origin in unfavourable cases (Fig. 57);

c) there is so far no unambiguous answer to the question whether more than one silver grain can form from a single silver halide crystal through photographical development;

d) a further factor bringing uncertainty is how far photographic development is extended to crystals which, while not latently exposed, are nevertheless in the immediate vicinity of the illuminated crystals; this factor commands caution in theoretical considerations.

Figs 57a to d give an idea of how the end product of the photographic process, the developed "grain" appears. As can be seen clearly, the form of the developed grains depends on the chemical composition of the developer. The absolute magnitude of the silver halide crystals is of only secondary importance for the appearance of the products of development. The figures illustrate the variety of possible grain forms encountered even with finer grain emulsions.

Concerning 3: Each β-particle liberated in radioactive decay receives a definite kinetic energy. The maximum path which can be covered with this energy, the range, depends on the initial energy of the emitted particle and on the medium in which the electron moves. There is no linear relation between the range and the radiation energy. On the contrary, the range increases more rapidly than would be anticipated from the energy increase. The dependence of the energy loss on the absolute value of the energy of the particle at the moment partially explains this observation (Chapter 2.). For example, if electrons of various energies traverse identical thicknesses of the same medium, each electron loses energy; but this energy loss on passing through the layer of medium is less, the higher the initial energy of the electron. Electrons of 10 keV lose on the average 150 eV in a 0.01 μ layer of a silver

* For further information, see H. Frieser, G. Haase and E. Klein: Grundlagen der photographischen Prozesse mit Silberhalogeniden, 3 volumes, Akad. Verlagsges. Frankfurt/Main, Germany 1968.

halide crystal; those of 100 keV lose only 17 eV [346]. In this case, thus, a tenfold increase in initial energy is accompanied by about a tenfold reduction in energy loss through traversing the same layer (Fig. 58). Each silver halide crystal needs a definite minimum energy

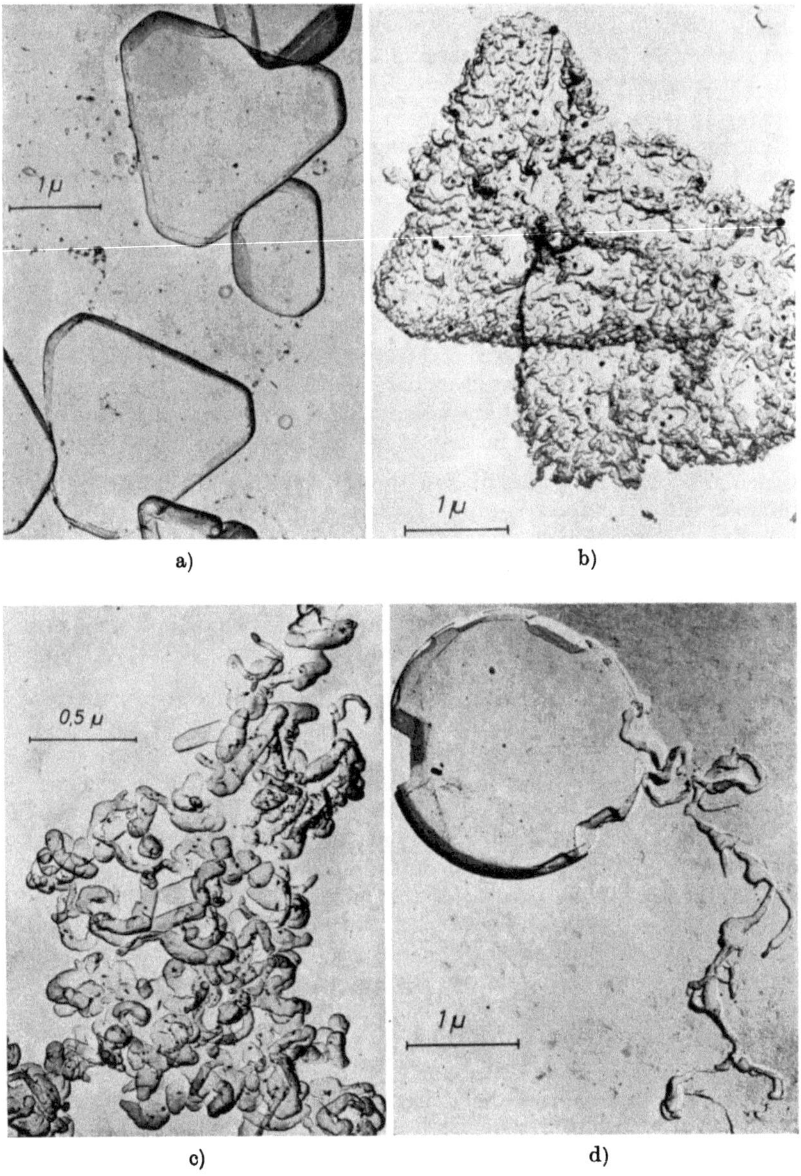

amount to bring it into a developable state. PELC, COOMBES and BUDD [347] give a figure of about 35 eV per grain. Since the energy given up depends on the existing energy of the particle, electrons of higher energy may thus bring about less exposure than the same number of electrons of lower energy on the same photographic layer. It is thus conceivable that electrons emerging from a source immediately below a silver halide crystal will not effect exposure of that grain because their energy is too high; they may, however, render developable more distant crystals which they reach after having lost energy. This could have a negative effect on the resolution of especially fine grain emulsions.

Concerning 4: Finally, in our opinion, the time of exposure has received too little attention in theoretical studies. For a qualitative treatment of the influence of exposure time on resolution, we will imagine the autoradiogram of an electron-microscope preparation which contains

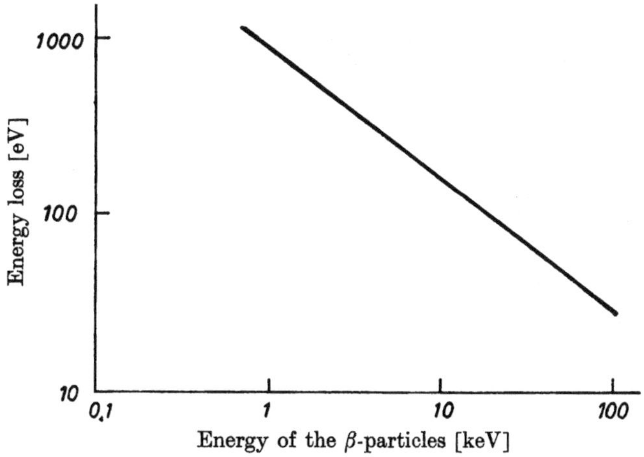

Fig. 58. Energy loss of β-particles while traversing a 100 Å layer of silver bromide, expressed as a function of their existing energy. According to PELC [346]

←

Fig. 57. Influence of the photographic development on the structure of the resulting silver. From KLEIN [232]

a) Carbon replica of the undeveloped silver halide crystal (From F. S. SJÖSTRAND: Electron Microscopy of Cells and Tissues, Acad. Press, N. Y., 1967, p. 417);
b) Product of development in a hydroquinone developer. The grain results in the same form and probably also in the same locality as the original crystal;
c) Bundle-shaped silver thread as a result of development in a p-phenylenediamine developer which is able to dissolve silver bromide;
d) Compact silver grain with attached thread. Physical developer. The origin of the development process cannot be located

several point sources of radiation. The space between adjacent sources shall be just large enough for each source to be distinguished or to be recognised from the autoradiogram, at least theoretically, based on the radiation distribution according to the RAYLEIGH criterion. It can be shown that, with present-day emulsions, the number of autoradiographic silver grains in the sphere of influence of each emitter is far too small for the position of the radiation sources to be clearly recognisable at any moment of autoradiographic exposure. Such distributions of blackening, corresponding to the radiation present above every individual source of radiation, cannot be realised within the relatively small region reached by the radiation on account of the size of the silver grains. If photographic development is begun early during exposure, there are too few silver grains to permit conclusions about a uniform distribution of activity in the preparation from the visible impression alone. One would naturally first conclude that the activity distribution was homogeneous when the autoradiogram is developed after extremely long exposure; all blackening differences are levelled by over-exposure, even those areas which have not been irradiated at all but have acquired a "background" value in the course of time. When discrete sources of radiation are present, a moment exists in the most favourable case between these extremes at which one can infer the position of the sources of radiation from the distribution of silver grains. Coordination of silver grains with the relevant sources of radiation is not possible merely through visual evaluation of the autoradiogram. Rather, an analysis of the distribution of grain density is necessary; a definite area is assumed around each grain in which the source of radiation is to be looked for. The time of exposure during which an analysis of this sort is possible depends on the intensity of radiation of the preparation. The higher this intensity is, the faster occurs the change over from the silver grain distribution at the outset to the renewed quasi-homogeneous distribution. This transition is critical because it can be effected through exposure of a fairly small number of silver halide crystals. This could be countered by trying to manage with lower activities so that a correspondingly longer time interval would be available for the change-over. This is only partially correct. The activity per layer is anyhow usually extremely low in electron-microscope autoradiography and the necessary times of exposure are exceedingly long.

The background value must not be neglected in considerations of exposure times. Long exposure times may mean appreciable background. This understandably affects adversely the interpretation of autoradiograms, the more so because discrete sources of radiation never occur in practice but only a more or less diffuse concentration of activity. According to our observations, it is impossible to decide whether a silver grain belongs to the background, already present, of an emulsion, or arises from radiation during exposure. Electron-microscope autoradiography can therefore be used rationally only when emulsions with negligible background are available. The interpretation of autoradiograms would be otherwise largely an arbitrary matter and in no way objective.

We have treated qualitatively here the difficulties of localisation in connection with the time of exposure, taking the example of discrete sources of radiation. We know of no publications in which the co-ordination problem has been quantitatively treated, taking into consideration the sensitivity to radiation of the emulsion, grain size, background and time of exposure. We have had to treat this problem exhaustively, however, in order to warn all those who are planning to use electron-microscope autoradiographic methods against exaggerated hopes and false conceptions.

Experience shows that it is at best possible with biological specimens to distinguish whether the active substance is in the nucleolus, on the nuclear membrane, in the cisterns of the endoplasmatic reticulum or in the mitochondria. One cannot distinguish with certainty between occurrence in the cristae or the mitochondria matrix (Reimer [VII]).

With regard to the practical evaluation of electron-microscope autoradiograms, it is helpful to have a direct measure of the distance around a silver grain in which the radioactive substance can be situated which was responsible for forming the grain. As our own investigations have shown [136], there is a rapid fall in the frequency with which silver grains are found in the vicinity of a tritium-containing preparation when

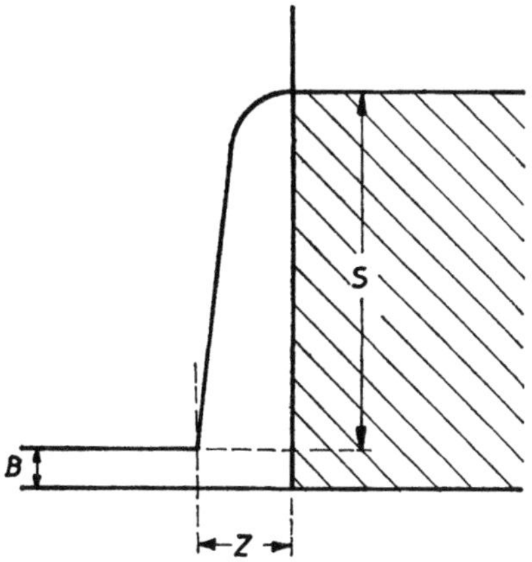

Fig. 59. Frequency of occurrence of silver grain during transition from the inactive to the active part of a monolayer preparation, according to Fischer and Werner [136]. The frequency (S) above the tritium-containing preparation falls to the value of the background (B) at a distance of 3 to 4 silver grain diameters (Z) from the radioactive preparation

the radioactive object is at a distance of about 3 to 4 silver grain diameters (Fig. 59). This observation agrees well with the previously given considerations on resolution and depicts the minimum uncertainty of electron-microscopic autoradiography. Recent experiments on resolution are quoted by SALPETER, BACHMANN and SALPETER [392].

6.3. Film material

One of the chief demands on the radiation-sensitive layer concerns the grain size of the emulsified silver halide crystals on which the resolution essentially depends (Section 6.2.). For some years, several emulsions have been available which can be used in electron-microscope autoradiography on account of their fine grain [162; 163; 488]. Their grain sizes and sensitivities to tritium β-radiation are summarised in Table 10.

The grain yields are given in the last column of Table 10. Some of the values have been taken from older work of various authors; differences from these may thus be found in later determinations. Incidentally, data often cannot be reproduced simply because of the fluctuating quality of different batches of the same emulsion material. Occasionally, traces of impurities suffice to change sensitivity markedly. Noteworthy is the comparatively high grain yield of emulsion types *NTE* and *NUC* which have the lowest average grain diameters. Sensitivity normally increases with increase in grain size, so that the finer grained emulsions should possess

Table 10

Grain diameter and sensitivity of some fine grain emulsions frequently used in high-resolution autoradiography

Emulsion	Grain diameter (Å)	Number of silver grains per tritium decay
Eastman-Kodak NTE*	300—500	1.30
Gevaert-Agfa NUC 3.07**	700	1.50
Ilford L4	1200	1.32
Gevaert-Agfa NUC 7.15**	1500	1.80
Ilford K 5	1800	1.00
Kodak V 1055	1700	0.51
Kodak AR 10	2000	0.57
Kodak NTA	2200	?
Eastman-Kodak NTB 3	2300	0.48
Eastman-Kodak NTB 2	2700	0.94

* data from SALPETER and BACHMANN [391].

** data from YOUNG and KOPRIWA [488]. All other data from CARO and VAN TUBERGEN [82].

the lowest sensitivities. The sensitivities of fine-grained emulsions have been brought into line with those of larger grain diameter by adding special sensitisers; these are added to the gelatine or adsorbed on the silver halide. A special part is played here by the ability of some substances to absorb radiation energy for short periods. The energy is stored in activated molecular states of short life. It is given up to the silver halide successively as low-energy quanta, yielding a larger number of latently exposed crystals than would be the case in the absence of these substances. The future of high resolution autoradiography perhaps lies in the development of still more effective sensitisers. An appreciable improvement of resolution and shortening of exposure time is imaginable with still finer-grained emulsions.

For use in electron-microscope autoradiography there are requirements of a photographic emulsion other than adequately fine grain and high sensitivity to radiation. Thus extremely thin films are needed for technical reasons in electron microscopy. Apart from the fact that the electron beam necessary for microscopy is usually absorbed already by very thin layers, the preparation warms up appreciably in the microscope during evaluation. It must thus be possible to work the film material into very thin layers and it must be thermally resistant so that it suffers no interfering changes during microscopy. In this latter context, practically only the gelatine is affected; silver grains could become embedded in it as a result of shrinkages. These effects have been successfully reduced to a minimum; yet one can observe with very fresh or also aged emulsions that the autoradiogram curls or even rolls up under the influence of the electron beam. A similarly undesirable effect is the loss of silver grains, presumably as a result of insufficient gelatine embedding. Such sites where silver grains formerly adhered can be recognised in the autoradiogram through the imprints remaining in the gelatine ("cats' footprints").

It is important in practice for the emulsion to show a high silver halide content from the beginning; or that this should be concentrated before use and should then be applied to the preparation with as uniform a grain distribution as possible. Methods for this are treated in the next section.

6.4. Description of some techniques

6.4.1. Preliminary note

Various techniques have been suggested for preparing and applying very thin layers of emulsion on to electron-microscopic preparations. There is no preferred method so far—proof that the methodological difficulties could not always be surmounted in the best way. Objective comparisons between different preparation techniques are also lacking. We are therefore restricting ourselves to acquainting the reader with a few published methods and to giving hints to help those interested in their choice of a suitable method.

6.4.2. Liquier-Milward's method

In the original form given here, Liquier-Milward's procedure [271] cannot be used in modern problems of histochemistry. The emulsion available at that time was too coarse and the film far too thick; at best, the attainable resolution would be equivalent to that of light-microscopic autoradiography. We are mentioning the procedure nevertheless because it represents the starting point in the development of electron-microscopic autoradiography and, in appreciably refined and modified form, formed the basis for development of subsequent procedures.
Ordinary glass slides were coated with a thin collodion or formvar film. The preparations to be autoradiographed were laid on the coated slides. Ilford *G5* emulsion was warmed to 50° C, diluted with water and allowed to drop on to the preparation. After drying, the whole was exposed in a light-tight, thick-walled lead container. After the autoradiographic exposure, development was carried out with the universal developer *D 19*, then fixing (2 min), washing (30 min) and drying. Finally the preparations plus attached film and autoradiogram were carefully detached from the slide and introduced on a suitable preparation holder into the electron microscope.
Fig. 60 shows an electron-micrograph of an autoradiogram obtained in this way. The origin of the radiation can be read from the clearly visible silver tracks.

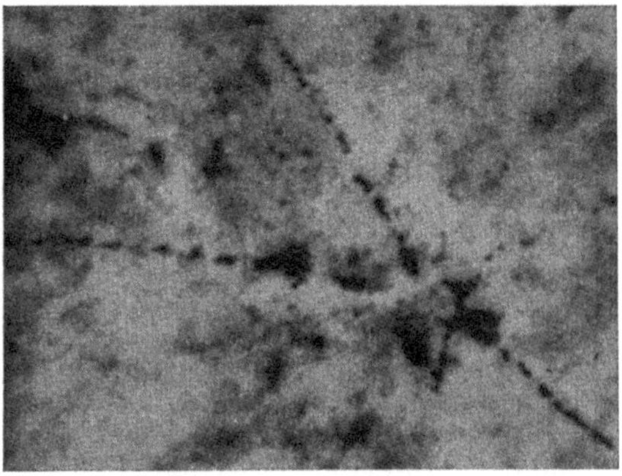

Fig. 60. Electron-micrograph (magnification ca 2,000 x) of a β-track autoradiogram. The radiation is emitted from tumour nuclei which had been labelled with ^{60}Co ($\beta_{max} = 0.3$ MeV). From [271]

6.4.3. Membrane method

Pelc, Coombes and Budd [347] first stretched formvar film over small plastic slides containing several bored holes of ca 7 mm diameter. The upper edge of each hole was smoothed to prevent damage to the membranes. Work was facilitated by fixing the plastic slides to a stand (Fig. 61). Thin sections, embedded in methacrylate or araldite, were mounted on the formvar membranes, accurately in the centre above each hole (Fig. 62).

Various radiation-sensitive emulsions, such as *G5*, *L4* (Ilford) or *NUC 3.07* (Gevaert-Agfa) were applied to the sections in red safelighting

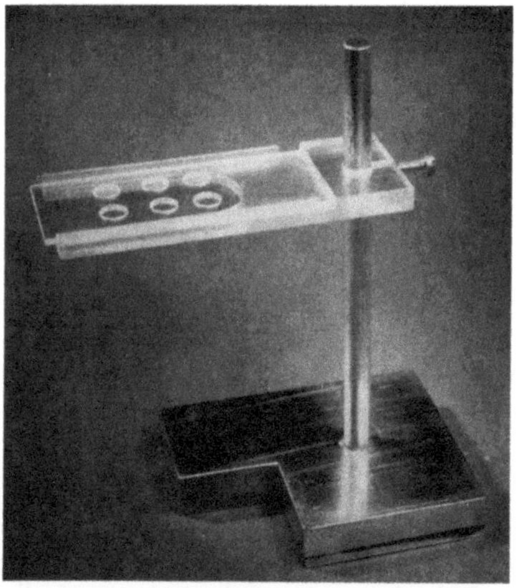

Fig. 61. Holder for plastic slides with holes (ca 7 mm diameter) in Pelc's membrane method. From [70]

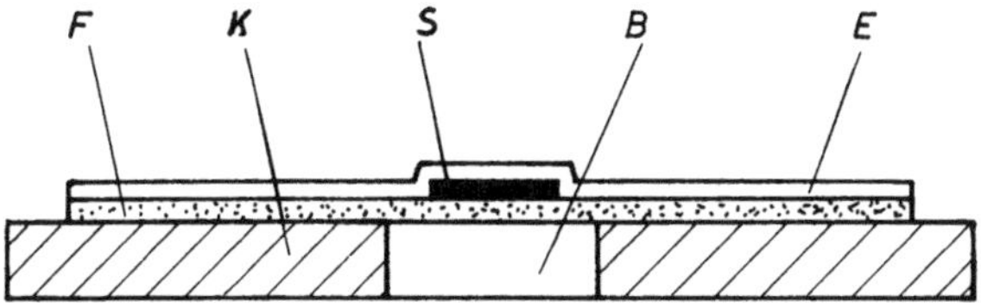

Fig. 62. Section through a preparation coated with emulsion according to Pelc, Coombes and Budd. B — hole, E — photographic emulsion, F — formvar membrane, K — plastic slide, S — thin section. After photographic development and contrast improvement, the specimen grid is pressed from below through the hole B on to the formvar membrane. The specimen-sandwich is then cut out with a scalpel

(*Wratten Filter, Series 1*). The emulsions had been previously warmed to 40 to 45°C and diluted with water in the ratio 1:5 or 1:10. One drop of the emulsion prepared in this way was placed on each section with a pipette and excess emulsion removed after 10 seconds. The emulsion still adhering to the preparation was dried for a few minutes at 45°C with the help of a hot plate. The dried preparations were exposed for up to 2 months in light-tight containers. After exposure, the autoradiograms were developed at 20°C in undiluted *D 19b* developer; 2 min was considered to be enough for this and also as the best as far as the silver grain size was concerned. The preparations were next briefly washed in distilled water and fixed for 5 minutes in a 20% sodium thiosulphate bath. Following this photographic development, the preparations can be treated with alkaline lead salt solutions or uranyl acetate to improve contrast. Finally, moistened specimen grids were pressed on to the under surface of the formvar membrane (likewise moistened with water); it was then carefully cut out around the grid [347; 70].

6.4.4. Methods with bubble-like emulsion lamellae

6.4.4.1. Principle

As has already been stated, high resolution is favoured if the preparation studied is coated as far as possible with only a single layer of thickly and uniformly packed silver halide crystals. In both the procedures described above (6.4.2. and 6.4.3.), control of the quality of the photographic layer is inadequate. The preparation of emulsion layers with reproducible thickness and crystal density is rendered more difficult by the influence of factors such as: degree of dilution; rate of sedimentation of the crystals; their adsorption on the surface of the preparation; rate of drying; air humidity; and the temperature dependence of all these. Many attempts have therefore been made to work out procedures which yield satisfactorily reproducible conditions [239]. The methods below depend on the idea of applying the principle of formation of soap lamellae; thin films of photographic emulsion are prepared by dipping rings and tubes in this manner. Amongst contributors may be mentioned: O'Brien and George II [325]; George II and Vogt [152]; Hampton and Quastler [180]; and Meek, Moses and Eiring [303].

6.4.4.2. The wire loop method

Caro and van Tubergen [82] described an original procedure for covering electron-microscope preparations with monolayers of the photographic emulsion *L4* (Ilford). At present it is the most widely used procedure, particularly in histoautoradiography. The method is suitable also for autoradiography of α- and proton radiation [269].

The emulsion, available in gel form, is first "thawed out" in the water bath at 45° C and diluted with distilled water; about 20 ml water and 10 g emulsion are mixed with a glass stirrer until homogeneous. The emulsion is cooled to room temperature within 2 to 3 minutes by adding ice to the water bath, so that it acquires the right viscosity for the application described below. After a further 30 minutes, the emulsion is viscous and ready for use. An oval platinum wire loop of 4 cm diameter is dipped into the emulsion and withdrawn slowly (copper wire loops, recommended as substitutes, are not advisable). If the emulsion has the correct consistency, a thin film is formed in the loop and immediately gelatinises.

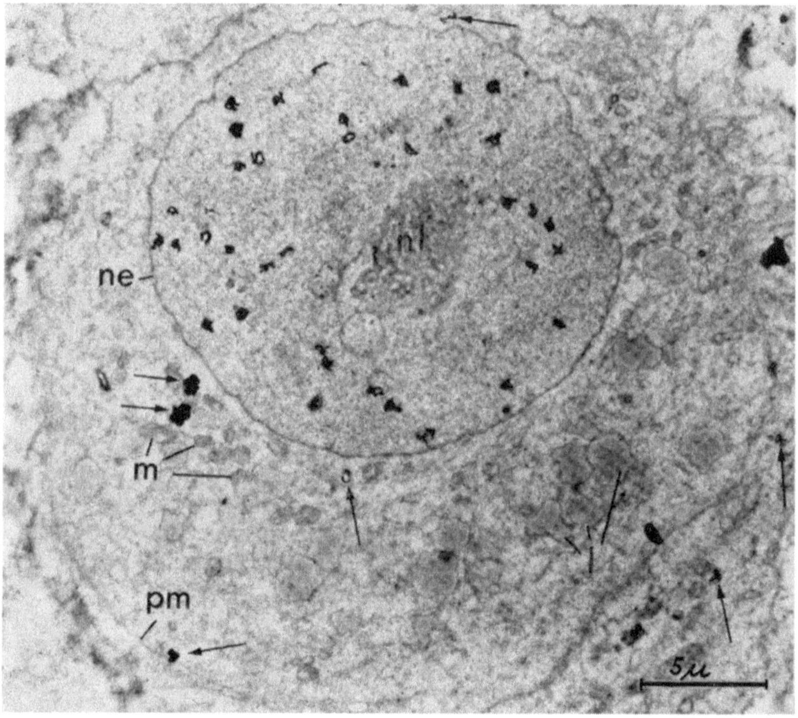

Fig. 63. Electron-microscopic autoradiogram of a *Hela* cell which had been treated 30 min earlier with the DNA precursor thymidine (labelled with tritium). From Moses [313].

The silver grains are distributed mainly over the nucleus, excepting the nucleolus (nl). Few grains appear in the vicinity of the nuclear membrane (ne), in the cytoplasm (arrows), near mitochondria (m) and on the plasma membrane (pm). *Ilford L4* emulsion, developed in *Microdol X* (5 min at 10° C); the preparation then treated with 0.02 N NaOH (30 min) and the contrast of the sections improved with 5% uranyl acetate (30 min)

The wire loop plus membrane is carefully laid on to the upper surface of a specimen grid which already carries the preparation to be autoradiographed. The emulsion membrane is detached from the loop when gently touched. It falls across preparation and slide and a very thin layer of emulsion remains adhering to the preparation.

This method has proved satisfactory in principle, yet its routine application is subject to certain difficulties. Thus, for example, the emulsion membrane may gelatinise too rapidly or collapse before being brought on to the specimen grid. Experience shows that freshly prepared batches of emulsion seldom yield good film layers. The membrane collapses often in the loop, especially with fresh preparations, before gel formation (recognisable through slight cloudiness) occurs at all. The strength of the film is claimed to be increased if the dilute emulsion is kept 10 to 12 hours at + 4°C in a refrigerator before being first used [340]. Only glass vessels must be used for preparing the emulsion. Moreover, the wall of the vessel in which the emulsion is warmed and diluted, should not come into contact with the stirrer during mixing. Friction between stirrer and wall can lead to reduction of silver halide and hence an increased background — possibly through local heating, electric discharge or triboluminescence.

The preparation of monolayers was improved materially by Haase and Jung [176]. They developed the wire loop method to the point where it can be applied to practically all photographic emulsions on the market. In their method, the emulsions are similarly warmed and diluted with distilled water so as to attain a suitable viscosity. Usually 4 to 6 parts of water are needed to accomplish this; some dilutions from the literature are in Table 11.

Table 11

Recommended dilutions of some emulsions for preparing monolayers by the wire loop method, as modified by Haase and Jung [176]

Emulsion	Dilution (Emulsion/water)	Authors
NTA (Kodak)	1 ml/2 ml	O'Brien, George [325] George, Vogt [152] Hampton, Quastler [180]
NTB 2 (Kodak)	1:1 to 1:10	Meek, Moses, Eiring [303] Meek, Moses [302]
L4 (Ilford)	1 g/2 ml 1 ml/7 ml	Caro, van Tubergen [82] Revel, Hay [362]
NUC 3.07 (Gevaert-Agfa)	1 g/0.6 g	Haase, Jung [176]
NUC 7.15 (Gevaert-Agfa)	1 ml/7 ml	Fromme [143]

In contrast to CARO and VAN TUBERGEN, the loops are not circular but have the elongated form seen in Fig. 64; this is claimed to achieve a better two-dimensional development of the monolayer within the emulsion membrane. In addition, a surface-active substance is added to the diluted emulsion to improve the surface tension property; e. g. *Hostapon T* (Farbwerke Hoechst AG, W. Germany) used as a wetting agent in the photographic trade. To obtain the desired viscosity at 30° C, it is best to add 3 to 5 drops of a ca 10% aqueous solution to 25 ml of the already diluted emulsion *NUC 3.07*. Especially stable *NUC*-monolayers, uniform and reproducible, are formed when the emulsion is first cooled at + 4° C for a few hours and then again warmed up to 30° C in the water bath. The area of monolayer within the loop (Fig. 64) becomes larger

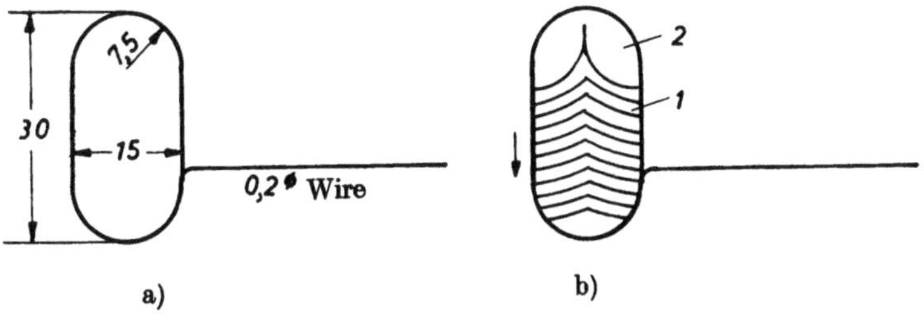

Fig. 64. Wire loop for preparing monolayers, according to HAASE and JUNG [176]
a) Suitable size; dimensions in mm;
b) Position of the interference bands [1] and the monolayer [2] in the gelatinised film layer. The emulsion thickens in the lower part of the loop. Gelatinisation begins at the topmost edge

when the loop is set up vertically after removing from the emulsion. When the wire loop is held so that the dark red light in the dark room shines through the membrane or is reflected, interference bands are seen which move upwards at the edge of the loop. The bands are a good indicator of the quality of the membrane. If they move upwards very rapidly, the emulsion is either too warm or too thin. Should the membrane burst quickly, the emulsion is allowed to stand some time outside the water bath until the movement of the bands has slowed up. On the other hand, with too cold or thick an emulsion, the bands quickly become motionless and the crystals will not be distributed homogeneously; the emulsion must then be warmed or diluted. It is advisable to hold the loop directly above the vessel containing the warmed emulsion. The lamella then dries or gelatinises substantially more slowly. No definite value for the best dilution of an emulsion can be given, since it appears to depend on the age and probably also on the varying nature of the gelatine from the different manufacturers [391].
A small, pale yellow zone is seen in daylight above the lower region of the loop characterised by the interference bands when Gevaert-Agfa

emulsion *NUC 3.07* is used. Haase and Jung showed that this was the site of the monolayer. This zone is described as gold coloured with the Ilford *L4* emulsion [340].
The film membrane is best applied by placing the specimen grids with the preparations on the upper flat ends of vertically fixed glass or plastic rods (Fig. 65). Holding the wire loop horizontally, the gelatinised membrane is brought carefully from above on to the preparation; one must ensure that only the monolayer zone comes into contact with the pre-

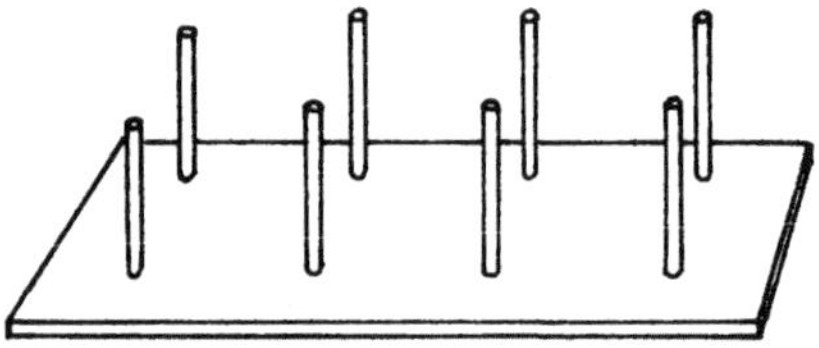

Fig. 65. A system of several rods, fixed to a common base, facilitates coating the specimen grids on the tops of the rods in the wire loop method

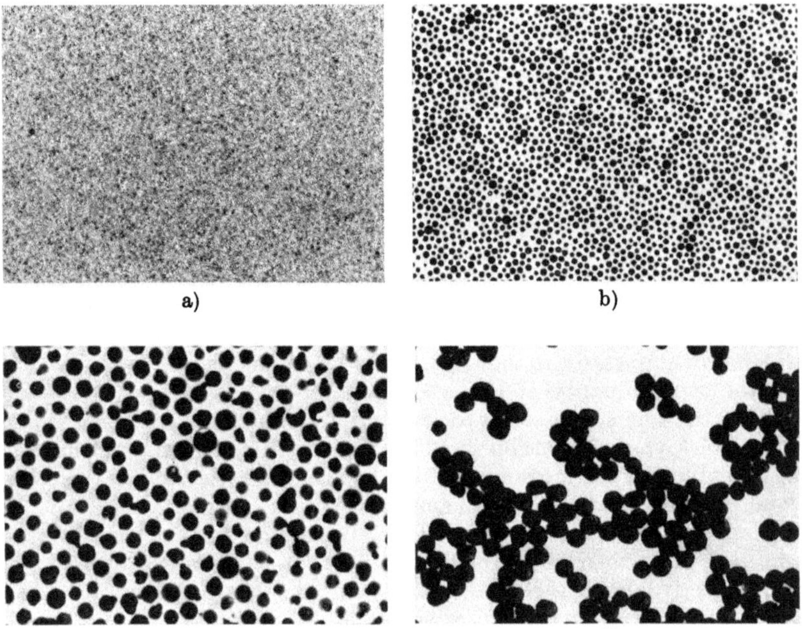

a) b) c) d)

Figs 66a, b and c. electron micrographs of a relatively well-formed monolayer from the "golden zone;" increasing magnification from a) to d).
d) monolayer outside the "golden zone;" large gaps are present between the irregularly distributed, clumped silver crystals

paration. This zone appears metallic silver-grey in the dark red light. All work with open emulsions naturally has to be carried out in the particular safety light recommended by the manufacturers. The freshly applied monolayer is said to adhere better to the preparation when briefly breathed on.

In our experience, HAASE and JUNG's modification of the method of CARO and VAN TUBERGEN offers the advantage of reproducible preparation of defined monolayers with comparatively little demands of time and technique. The photographic development of the exposed preparations presents no particular difficulties (see Section 6.6,).

6.4.4.3. The bubble method

In order to prepare thin monolayers more uniform and perfect than film layers made by the various other procedures known at that time, CARO [76] likewise utilised the ability of gelatinous emulsions to form skin-like lamellae. His procedure differs from the wire loop method described above, in which the emulsion membrane at least partly runs into a monolayer under the influence of the surface tension and probably also as a result of differences in density between the silver halide crystals and the gelatine; he tried preparing bubbles to achieve homogeneous distribution of the silver halide and to thin the emulsion layer.

5 g of Ilford *K5* emulsion are warmed to 45°C in a water bath with 40 ml of 0.1% aqueous KBr solution and mixed well with a glass stirrer. As a result of capillary attraction, a small amount of this solution rises

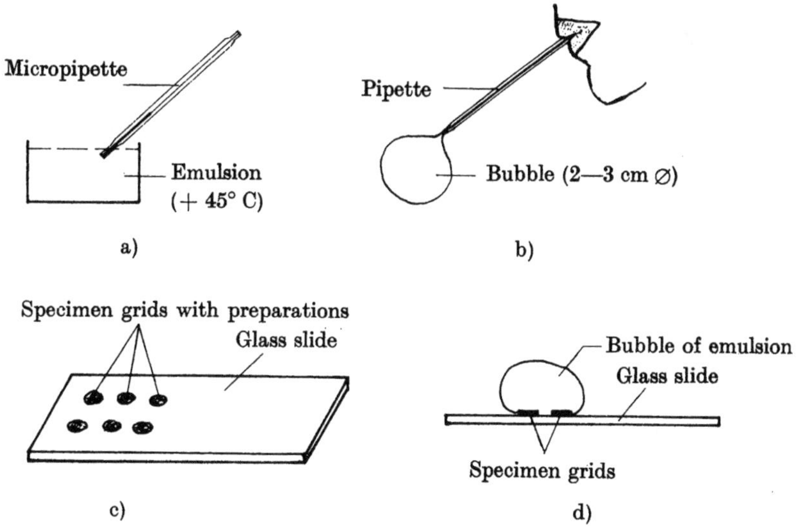

Fig. 67. Bubble method of CARO [76]; details in text

into a micropipette dipped into it. An emulsion bubble of about 2 cm diameter can be fashioned from this small amount by carefully blowing air from the mouth. Caro transfers the bubble on to glass slides, pretreated with 0.1% gelatine and 0.01% chrome alum and on which were situated specimen grids carrying preparations (Fig. 67). To prevent the grids from slipping during this working operation, they are secured to the glass slide at a corner well away from the preparation, using a trace of adhesive (rubber cement). After the bubble bursts, a thin uniform layer of emulsion should spread over the part of the glass slide carrying the specimen grid. Emulsion drying is accelerated by passing dry air over it. During autoradiographic exposure, the preparations are kept by Caro on the glass slide at + 4°C in closed containers under CO_2 and in presence of a drying agent. Photographic development is in *D19* (Kodak), lasting 2 minutes; fixing takes 5 minutes and after briefly washing in running distilled water, contrast may be improved by 10 minutes treatment with 1% uranyl acetate in 50% alcohol. The specimen grids are then carefully separated from the glass.

We know of no literature references to a more extensive application of the bubble method.

6.4.4.4. Other procedures with emulsion lamellae

A procedure in which the emulsion membrane is used before it gelatinises is due also to Caro and van Tubergen [82]. It is relatively involved, the more so because all the more difficult operations have to be carried out in the dark room.

A membrane is fashioned on the bottom of a petri dish from a 2% aqueous agar solution. It is then dried out completely and stored in a refrigerator. Rectangular pieces, about 2 × 3 cm, are cut out of it and laid on ordinary glass slides. The surface of the agar membrane which was in contact with the bottom of the petri dish faces upwards, away from the glass slide. The agar rectangles are soaked with 0.2% collodion solution in amyl acetate and dried in a vertical position. An Ilford *L4* emulsion membrane is now made with the help of a loop as described in Section 6.4.4.2.; before it gelatinises, it is brought on to the collodion-agar surface. Since the surface is even and drying of the emulsion is favoured through the adjoining membrane, a highly uniform emulsion skin with homogeneous distribution of silver salt is claimed to be formed. The collodion-emulsion double membrane is transferred to a water surface with the emulsion skin uppermost. Finally, preparations supported on specimen grids are brought from underneath on to the floating membrane and withdrawn from the water. The preparations are thus in direct contact with the collodion layer which separates them from the emulsion. After drying, exposure is carried out at + 4°C.

This interposed barrier of a collodion membrane between preparation and radiation-sensitive layer necessarily reduces the resolution and also

the number of lower-energy ß-particles which would normally reach the photographic layer. A compensating advantage is that chemographic effects from the preparation are suppressed.
Apart from these methods just described, there are still further variations for preparing monolayers and for bringing these on to electron-microscopic preparations with the aid of the wire loop method [288].

6.4.5. Dipping procedures

According to HAY and REVEL [185; 363], FEWER et al [131] and KOPRIWA [239], procedures for preparing sufficiently thin and uniform photographic layers on electron-microscopic preparations can be based on the *dipping* procedure [305] of ordinary light-microscopic autoradiography (Section 5.3.); this involves simple immersion in a "melted" and, if necessary, diluted photographic emulsion.
HAY and REVEL attach the specimen grid + preparation to be coated with emulsion to glass slides by means of adhesive tape on both sides. These are then dipped into Ilford *L4* emulsion-distilled water (1 + 7 to 8) and suspended vertically to dry. Autoradiographic exposure is performed at + 4° C and is followed by developing the grids, still fixed to the glass slides, for 2 minutes in *Dektol* (Kodak)-water (1 + 2) and then fixing for 5 minutes. The contrast of the still moist preparations is improved for electron microscopy by KARNOVSKI lead staining. The photographic gelatine layer is too thick for electron microscopy and most of it is then removed with 0.02M NaOH.
PRZYBYLSKI'S procedure [354] is similar. He attaches his preparation grids to glass slides also with adhesive tape but applies the emulsion of Ilford *G5*-water (1 + 15) at 45° C with a camel hair brush.
All these methods have the shortcoming that the specimen grids do not acquire a homogeneous coating because the emulsion does not dry uniformly. This shows up as an enrichment of silver halide on the grid wires. KOPRIWA [238] tried to avoid this by using a semi-automatic device for coating the grids. Glass slides are first coated with celloidin. They are then placed in an automatically driven dipping contrivance and immersed in the particular emulsion under absolutely reproducible conditions; the optimum dilution of each emulsion is established previously. Speed of immersion and withdrawal can be varied (Fig. 68). After the emulsion has dried, small 3 × 3 mm squares are scratched into it, floated on to the surface of distilled water and transferred to specimen grids on which the preparations are already situated.
SALPETER and BACHMANN [391] first mount the thin sections on glass slides coated with a film of collodion. They then deposit a layer of carbon and drop on emulsion at 60° C. Any excess is absorbed with filter paper. Drying is again in the vertical position. After exposure, the preparations are photographically developed on the glass slides and then floated off in

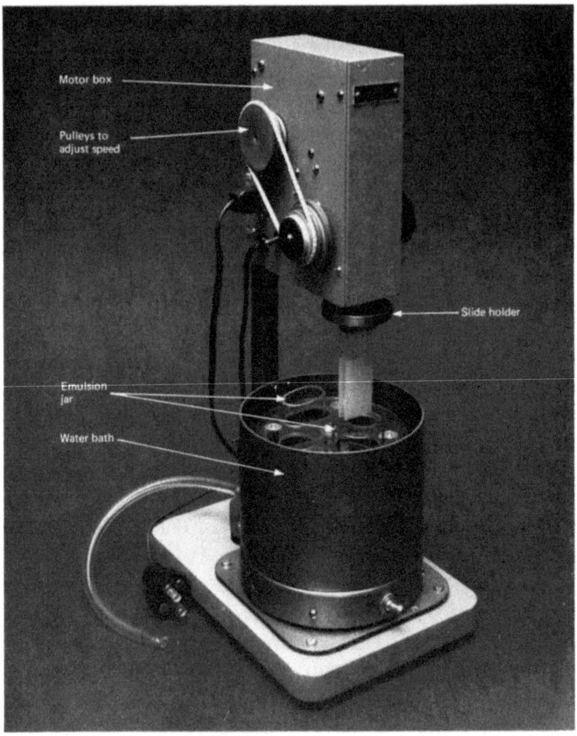

Fig. 68. Apparatus for coating slides with a uniform layer of emulsion, according to Kopriwa [239]

water. The autoradiogram remains adhering to the preparation. Specimen grids are placed over the preparations and the complete sandwich is lifted from the water surface with filter paper in the usual way (Fig. 69).

Bachmann and Salpeter [21; 22; 23] used also the very fine grained emulsion *NTE* (Eastman Kodak) as well as *L4* (Ilford). The former has some advantages over the frequently used latter, due to undeveloped *NTE*-grain having a diameter of only 300 to 500 Å. The commercially available form of the emulsion, however, contains excess gelatine for reasons of stability; the photographically effective components must therefore be concentrated before use. To this end, one adds 10 ml distilled water to each gram *NTE* and warms the mixture to 60° C on a water bath, stirring cautiously. The excess of water-soluble gelatine is separated with a laboratory centrifuge, kept at about 40° C with a stream of warm air (hair drier). Before the supernatant is separated, the sediment is cooled for about 20 seconds in ice water. Two further 1 ml portions of

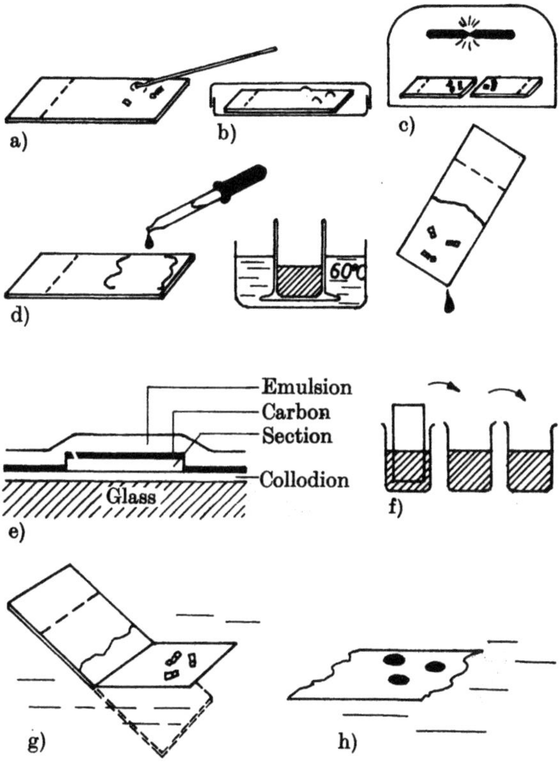

Fig. 69. Preparation of electron-microscopic autoradiograms according to Salpeter and Bachmann [391]; details in text

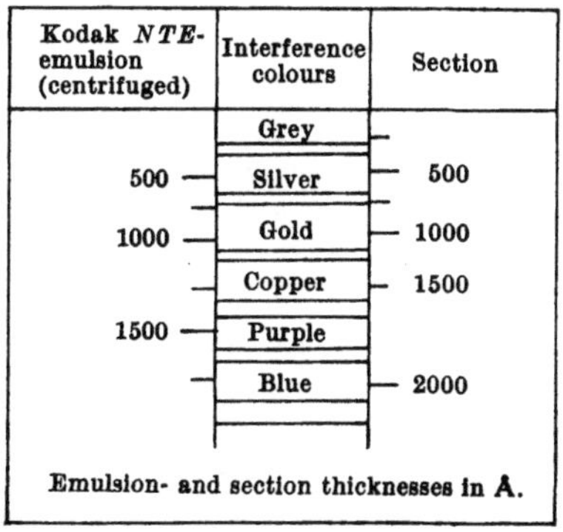

Fig. 70. Estimation of the thickness of embedded histological thin layer preparations and of fine-grained photographic emulsions, based on their interference colours; according to Salpeter and Bachmann [391]

water are added and the mixture centrifuged each time as described to concentrate further. All these operations must naturally be carried out in safety light, e. g., *Wratten OA* (Kodak). The correct concentration can be recognised from the interference colour of an emulsion layer prepared by placing a drop on to a glass slide and holding this vertically until the emulsion which does not run off, dries. A *NTE* monolayer is said to appear silver to pale gold in daylight when it is 600 Å thick (Fig. 70).

6.4.6. Centrifuge methods

Koehler, Mühlethaler and Frey-Wyssling [235] were dissatisfied with the results of the above-mentioned techniques for applying emulsion and proposed another way: Electron-microscope preparations, coated with carbon by vapour deposition, on specimen grids are carefully placed with the carbon layer downwards on a floating formvar film. This is best performed by grouping several grids closely together so that they, together with the adhering formvar film, can be easily lifted from above with sintered glass

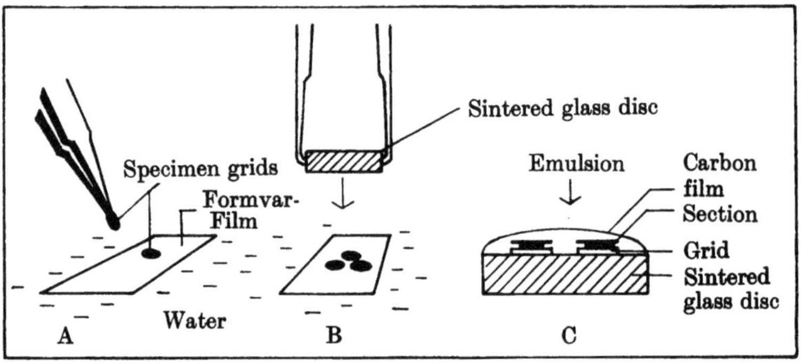

Fig. 71. Preparation of specimens for electron-microscope autoradiography according to Koehler et al [235]. Specimen grids with carbon-vaporised preparations are laid on floating formvar film (A) and the whole is lifted from the water surface (B, C)

filter discs (Fig. 71). The "sandwich", consisting of formvar film, carbon layer, thin section, specimen grid and sintered glass disc, is placed exactly in the centre of the rotating head of a laboratory centrifuge containing a suitable sized depression in which the sintered glass disc fits (Fig. 72). The formvar film, situated uppermost, serves to provide a uniformly smooth and plane base for the emulsion which is dropped on to it and dispersed through centrifugal force. The authors use the Ilford *G5* emulsion at 45°C, previously diluted 1:1 with distilled water. One to two drops of this diluted emulsion are dropped from a height of 5 cm on to the sintered disc, rotating at 10,000 rpm. The emulsion thereby runs into a uniform layer without the crystals forming a density gradient or the layer thickness depending on the distance from the axis of rotation. This effect appears at first sight to contradict the centrifugal principle. It may perhaps be explained by gelatinisation of the emulsion during centrifuging, so that the crystals are "frozen" and prevented from further radial displacement. After applying the emulsion, one should always study an undeveloped test preparation to check density and distribution of the silver bromide crystals. Circumstances can be modified if necessary by varying the emulsion dilution or speed of revolution of the centrifuge.

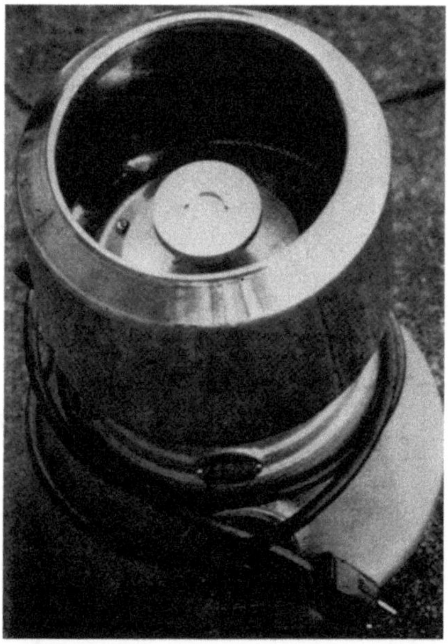

Fig. 72. Centrifuge with depression in the rotating head to take a sintered glass disc; according to KOEHLER et al [235]. Details in text

KOEHLER et al undertake autoradiographic exposure and subsequent photographic development with the sintered glass disc present. The time of development in *D 19b* developer-water (1 + 1) is 1 minute and fixing time is 2 to 3 minutes.

ROHR, KLIETMANN and OEHLERT [375] also prepared autoradiograms by a procedure based on that reported here. However, they used a centrifuge head made of plastic, in which a circular dental wax form was let in. Two or three copper grids were mounted slightly excentrically in small indentations of the plate.

ROHR et al developed according to data of CARO and VAN TUBERGEN [82] and GRANBOULAN et al [164]. One litre of the aqueous developer solution contains:

2 g *ecol*(p-methylaminophenol sulphate)
40 g sodium carbonate
100 g sodium sulphite
1 g potassium bromide.

This solution is placed in a developing dish and the wax plates with the film-coated, ultra-thin sections laid on the surface of the solution so that section faces solution. Development is for 2 minutes. Without rinsing with water, the wax plates are then fixed for 10 minutes in a sodium thiosulphate bath in the same position. The preparations are briefly but carefully washed with water and contrast improved by the KARNOVSKI lead procedure in the usual way and without prior drying. The staining solution is diluted 1:50 and the procedure lasts 30 to 60 minutes at + 4°C.

DOHLMAN et al [106; 105] describe another method for preparing uniform monolayers of silver bromide crystals using a centrifuge. They place copper grids, coated with formvar, in Plexiglas* holders expressly designed for insertion in glass centrifuge tubes (Fig. 73). The grids are

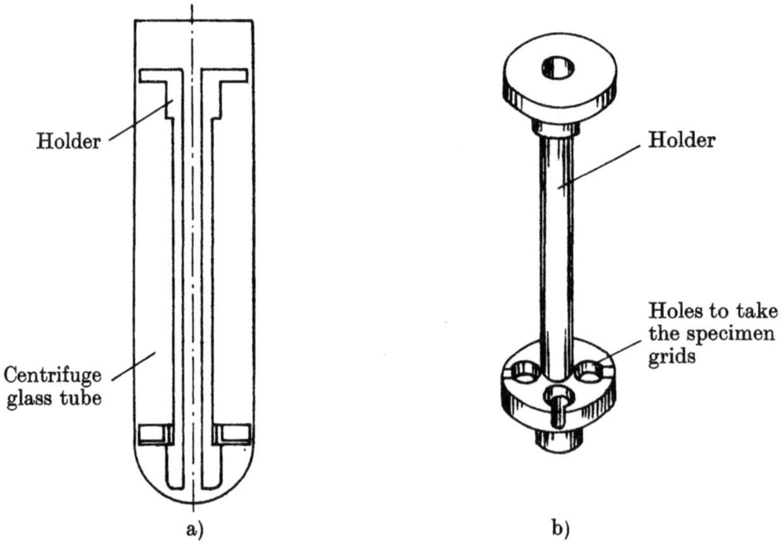

Fig. 73. Preparation of monolayers according to DOHLMAN et al [106]
a) Centrifuge tube with Plexiglas* holder (section along its length);
b) Plexiglas* holder with holes for taking the grids

* Polymethyl methacrylate, resembling Perspex.

carefully fixed with a trace of rubber solution above the holes at the lower end of the holder. Ilford *L2* emulsion is diluted in the ratio 1g:15 litres water and the centrifuge tube half filled with this solution. This is centrifuged for 5 min at 500g. Heavier conglomerates are thereby precipitated and only then is the accurately fitting Plexiglas holder with specimen grids introduced into the centrifuge glass. The holes beneath the grids are previously filled with distilled water to avoid interference by ascending air bubbles. The diluted, precentrifuged emulsion must extend up to 20 mm above the grids. This is centrifuged for 10 minutes at 10,000 rpm, corresponding to about 10,000 g with respect to the grids. 0.5 ml of 40% formalin solution or a little absolute alcohol is added dropwise to the hole in the longitudinal axis of the holder before taking it out of the centrifuge tube (Fig. 73). This is stated to stabilise mechanically the sedimented layer grain. The emulsion-coated preparations are left to air-dry. Coating with a thin collodion membrane is recommended to protect the photographic layer and to prevent silver grains from displacement during photographic development. Development and fixing of the autoradiograms was performed with, respectively, Kodak developer *D 19b* (5 minutes) and *G305-A-fixative* (10 minutes). All work was carried out in the safety light from the *Kodak Wratten Filter OB.*

6.4.7. Nuclear-track microautoradiography

A method of RIEDEL [365] is less suitable for autoradiography of biological specimens than for studies of radioactive dusts or aerosols. A "noodle" of nuclear track emulsion, Ilford *L4*, is placed in a dropping bottle in red light in the dark room, warmed to 35°C in a thermostat and kept until completely "melted." A small amount is then dropped on to a 7 × 10 cm glass plate. This is spread uniformly to give the desired thickness over the whole plate, using a "Lackhantel" (a type of rolling pin*). 40 drops of emulsion yield a microlayer of film of about 90 μ; this shrinks to about one-tenth of this thickness on drying. Radioactive preparation and microlayer are united just before the surface of the emulsion, sticky for a long period, has dried out. With aerosol preparations, the membrane filter carrying the sample is simply pressed against the emulsion layer and then carefully removed. When circumstances permit, the sample can also be floated in water and drops brought on to the emulsion in a very finely divided state as a hydrosol, using an electric sprayer. The fast moving particles lose water in flight as a result of its high vapour pressure, and adhere especially firmly to the emulsion. The film is finally scarified with a "Gitterschnittprüfer"* and photographically developed. At the end, the small squares of film are floated off and these are taken up with the usual specimen grids for electron

* Firm of Retsch, Haan, W. Germany.

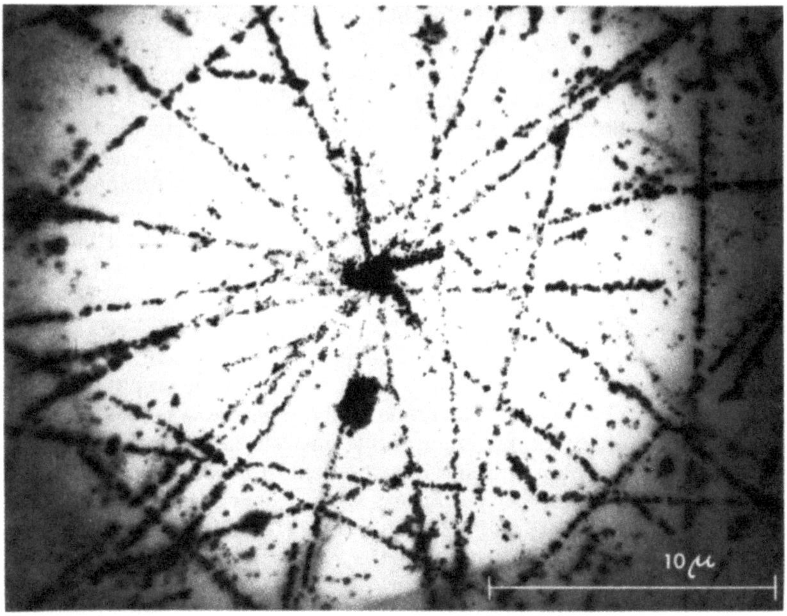

Fig. 74. Tracks emanating from radioactive dust particles. RIEDEL's method [365]

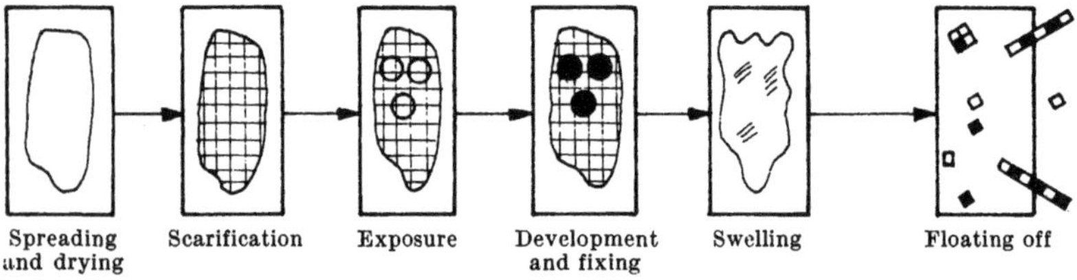

Fig. 75. Scheme for preparing nuclear track films due to RIEDEL [365]

microscopy (Fig. 75). As a result of the scarification, a 2 mm margin along the length of the emulsion layer suffers latent exposure; this can be recognised as a black frame to the otherwise transparent emulsion when each square is floated.

6.5. Other techniques; prospect of newer developments

SILK et al [414] tried out a new type of method for obtaining monolayers of high density. The principle of the method is the vapour deposition of silver at 10^{-4} mm Hg on to the electron-microscope preparation, situated on a grid with a formvar film. The silver layer, 150 to 450 Å thick and consisting of a conglomeration of tiny silver crystallites growing together, is exposed to bromine vapour. Within only 2 minutes, the light silver-coloured preparation becomes covered with a white layer of silver bromide. This is subsequently stabilised with a film of gelatine. The grain size of the silver bromide is given as 250 to 1100 Å. Work must be performed in a dark room from the moment of bromination. The Agfa safety filter *L 107* provides suitable illumination.

The vapour deposition technique has not proved satisfactory. The very low sensitivity of the film to radiation may be given as chief reason; this results from the especially fine grain. The dense crystal layer is also a disadvantage. The photographic development process does not stop at the boundaries of the grains but may extend via many crystals since these are often too close to one another and can be "infected" during the development. The advantage of high resolution which had been hoped for from the silver vapour deposition technique has not materialised [346].

Attempts were made to improve resolution in light-microscope autoradiography by impregnating the specimens with silver salts [411; 412]. Although these techniques have made no breakthrough, the possibility of a successful revival in electron-microscope autoradiography remains. It has not been possible so far to apply them with preparations made through embedding in plastic. Silver impregnation should, however, be compatible with the ultra-thin freeze-sectioning technique which has been coming into use lately, provided that chemography can be prevented. Homogeneous saturation of preparations with silver salts will not be fully realisable as a result of obstacles related to structure. The consequences of this will affect quantitative autoradiography first and foremost.

Another attempt is in the direction of completely abandoning any photographic layer situated directly on the preparation. Strictly speaking, this principle has nothing more to do with autoradiography. It depends on using a special electron microscope to detect the ß-particles being emitted from a radioactively labelled preparation. The β-particles liberated in the decay are shown up on a fluorescent screen or immediately recorded on film material. A highly magnified "autoradioscintogram" is yielded; this can be subsequently coordinated without difficulty with an electron-micrograph of the particular specimen detail, taken on the same scale. Before the experiments of LIQUIER-MILWARD, the founder of electron-microscope autoradiography, devices of this sort had been tested out in fact by MARTON and ABELSON [295] and by BARKER, RICHARDSON and FEATHER [26]. At that time, however, the sensitivity of the technical procedures was too low, even at relatively high activities; only monoenergetic β-particles could be utilised. Since most emitters have a continuous and not monoenergetic β-spectrum, further efforts in this field are concentrating on constructing an acrhomatic, spherically corrected electron optical system, available for all energy regions. The question remains whether it is worth the outlay of time and technique compared with the "classical" electron microscopy with silver halides. The preparation of a single autoradiogram would keep an electron microscope occupied perhaps for several weeks on this alone, merely to establish ultimately that, for example, a particular cell nucleus of interest is totally unlabelled. On the other hand, a device of this sort offers the possibility of pursuing autoradiographic, kinetic *in-vivo* studies — e. g. following directly the transport route of a radioisotope in the intracellular region. Plans of this sort belong at the moment to the realm of fantasy.

Direct utilisation of a magnetic field seemed more profitable to some authors. HARFORD and HAMLIN [183; 182] published in 1961 work in which they claimed that the field of a permanent magnet influences grain yield. According to their studies, a marked increase in the number of silver grains over the radioactive areas of a preparation is to be expected in a magnetic field of 10^4 gauss. Control preparations, exposed outside the magnetic field, showed altogether fewer silver grains and relatively intense background which interfered considerably with evaluation. Further, the form of the developed silver filaments in the two cases was said to differ characteristically. These results have been accepted generally with some scepticism. In CARO's opinion [75], the increase in yield cannot be explained through the typical screw-like movement of free electrons in a magnetic field. For example, electrons of 10 keV possess an orbit of 680 μ diameter in a magnetic field of 10^4 gauss. The maximum range of tritium β-particles is only 2.5 μ in fine-grained emulsions. Fields of the order of 10^6 gauss would be necessary to force electrons emitted at an acute angle to the plane of the section, into and through the emulsion; this would effect an appreciable improvement in autoradiographic resolution. At the present time, such fields can be prepared only for microseconds. FROMME and ZESSACK [145] commented similarly on the results discussed above. They also could find no experimental differences between exposures within and outside a magnetic field. On the other hand, NAKAI [317] obtained a marked rise in the autoradiographic silver grains during exposure in a static magnetic field, the strength of which he did not quote. He worked with ^{35}S-labelled substances. Although the maximum range of ^{35}S β-radiation is even about ten times greater than that of tritium, resolutions near to the theoretical limit of ca 1000 Å (see Section 6.2.1.) were claimed. NAKAI's preparations were made by a method based on that of PRZYBYLSKI (see 6.4.5.). As shown in Fig. 76, they were fastened to glass slides with adhesive tape and exposed on the poles of a powerful horseshoe magnet in the dark at ca + 4° C for up to two months. The author, aware of the previously mentioned critical attitude to exposure in a magnetic field, can offer no explanation for the higher silver grain yield.

MIZUHIRA [309], MIZUHIRA and UCHIDA [310] and TER-POGOSSIAN, DONADIEU, MORENO and BESSIS [440] have recently rekindled discussion

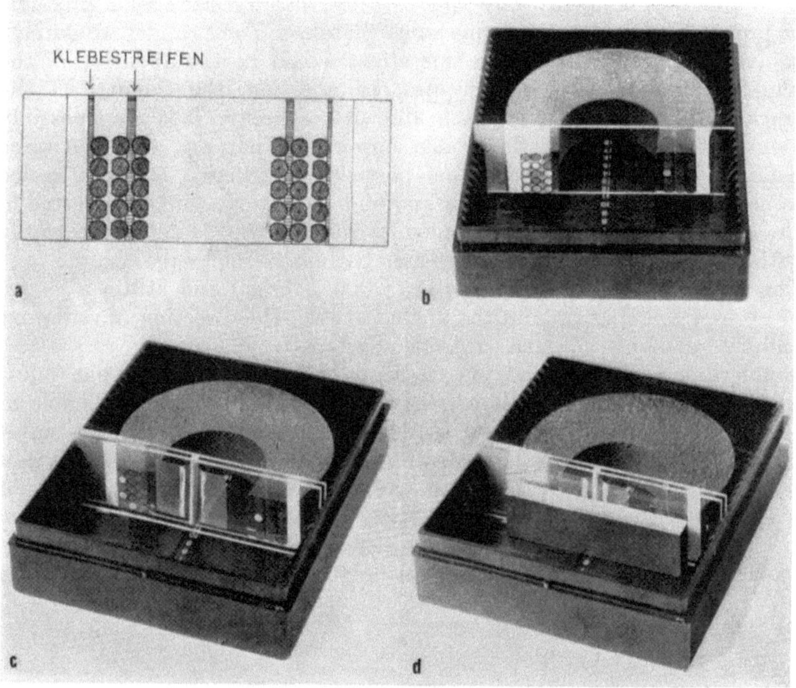

Fig. 76. Exposure in a magnetic field according to NAKAI [317]
The specimen grids, coated with emulsion, were attached to glass slides according to PRZYBYLSKI's method [354] (a). The preparations were laid on the poles of a horseshoe magnet (b) and were covered with another slide (c). The magnetic field was intensified with an armature (d)
Klebestreifen = Adhesive tape

of this theme.They observed a positive influence of exposure in a magnetic field on resolution and grain yield. Should these results prove to be reproducible and not random, insignificant, single data, one ought to devote special attention to the magnetic field, at least from the point of view of scientific photography. It is a fact that such effects cannot be explained alone through a change of path of the β-particles.

It is remarkable that there have so far been no publications on the use of electric fields for improving autoradiographic resolution; the principle of exposure in an electric field was the subject of a patent some time ago [210].

The attempt to replace silver salts by other substances as radiation detectors represents another development connected with electron-microscope autoradiography. Physically homogeneous layers are aimed at, in order to circumvent difficulties arising out of the inhomogeneous emulsions of suspended crystals [17].

Silk and Barnes [413] were able to show that nuclear fission products of uranium leave tracks in fine mica platelets. The primary advantage of autoradiography based on this effect would be the abolition of the photographic development process. In addition, the fineness of the tracks aid coordination of track and site of decay. This may possibly yield better resolution. It is also important that one and the same medium is suitable for recording particles of differing energies in the same way. Radiation of both low and high energy can thus be detected in the same specimen and reasonable electron-microscope autoradiography with emitters of higher energy than tritium becomes possible at last. The tracks in the mica are less than 300 Å broad and attain a length of up to 4 μ, depending on the angle between the direction of radiation and the plane of the mica (Fig. 77).

Metal films [323; 50] and plastic films [282; 283; 92] are, like mica, suitable for registering fission fragment tracks. Although applicable in theory, these techniques have scarcely been used up to now for autoradiography of biological preparations. An example is due to Malmon [283] who treated viruses with uranyl acetate containing 93% of ^{235}U isotope. This introduced about 3 uranium atoms per virus, an extremely small uptake. The viruses were then prepared for electron-microscopic inspection and the preparations submitted to thermal neutrons

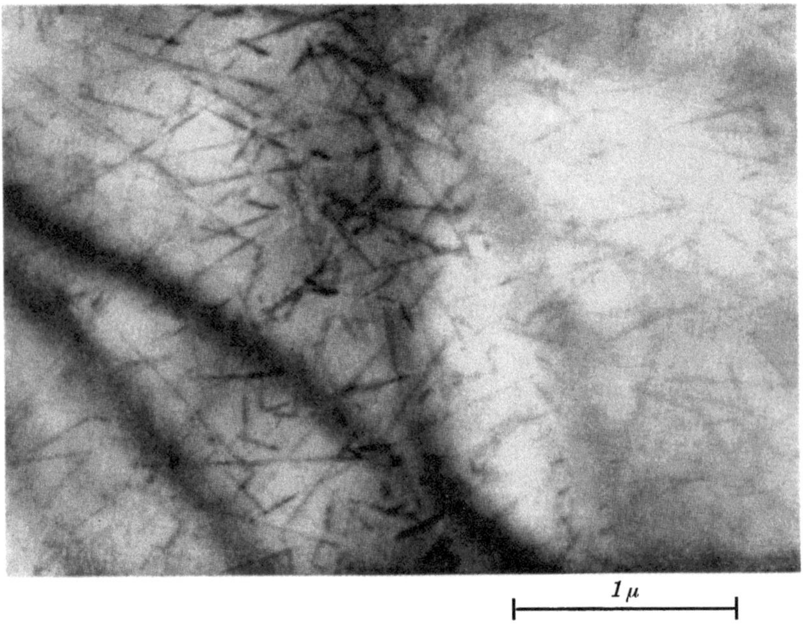

Fig. 77. Tracks of uranium fission products in a mica platelet, from Silk and Barnes [413]

in the reactor. This brought about nuclear fission of the ^{235}U. Layers of chromium, platinum, platinum-palladium and silicon monoxide were tested as detectors for these fission products. Chromium films of 50 to 100 Å thickness proved to be the best. The position of individual uranium atoms on the DNA-strand was said to be determinable with an accuracy of 50 Å. We are dealing here with the absolutely most sensitive autoradiographic method which we know of, both with regard to the low rate of uptake and on account of the extremely high resolution. Even single atoms can be detected. Unfortunately its application is restricted to the uranium isotope ^{235}U which can be artificially split by neutrons.

The interesting use of plastic films to detect α-particles is due likewise to MALMON [284]. These α-particles arise from ^{17}O through bombardment with thermal neutrons and from ^{15}N and ^{18}O through irradiation with protons. A new prospect for biochemistry and histochemistry arises from the possibility of introducing such elements, although they possess no utilisable radioactive isotopes.

Shorter autoradiographic exposure times without detrimental effect on resolution can be achieved by incorporating a scintillator (such as "PPO") into the embedding media. This modification may also increase the number of radioactive isotopes that up to now could be used for autoradiographic studies*.

6.6. Autoradiographic exposure of electron-microscope specimens

Exposure times in electron-microscopic autoradiography are necessarily longer than in autoradiography of macroscopic and light-microscopic specimens. This is due to the high magnification at which electron-microscope autoradiograms are evaluated; to the activity applicable to a specimen under examination; to the very small mass of the preparations compared to the original specimen; and to the small silver grain yield (averaging 1 grain per electron). This in turn requires factors to be considered which are of subsidiary importance in "normal" autoradiography. For example: the stability of a latent image or the change with time of properties specific to the emulsion, especially sensitivity to radition, background, stability and demands on photographic development. These factors have been the object of numerous studies, all the data and results of which cannot be generalised since they refer to particular emulsions or autoradiographic techniques. We wish to summarise below some generally useful knowledge [136]:

1. Every photographic emulsion possesses a background from the moment of its preparation. It is of the order of 10^6 to 10^7 grains/cm^2.

* FISCHER, A. H., H. KORR, H. THIELE and G. WERNER: Naturwissenschaften **58** (1971) 101.

2. The background increases with increasing age and therefore also during autoradiographic exposure. This increase depends on temperature. The increase at lower temperatures is usually small.
3. Unless the manufacturer recommends otherwise and the preparations tolerate it, photographic emulsions and undeveloped, emulsion-coated preparations should be stored in a refrigerator at temperatures above 0° C, at ca +4° to +6° C.

Apart from the favourable influence of temperatures around 0° C in suppressing background, regression of the latent image also depends on temperature. This is termed *fading*. It increases at higher temperature, thus showing a temperature variance in the same sense as background growth. It is an irreversible process and a loss of latent image, once it has occurred, cannot be reversed photochemically. Fading is, chemically, oxidation of the minute traces of silver which outline the latent image. Hitherto there have been few quantitative studies of the fading effect [337; 444; 468]. Its significance in autoradiography thus cannot yet be perceived. The methods used in practice to suppress fading are therefore only empirically based [78]. Moreover, the time-dependence of the regression of the latent image fluctuates sharply from emulsion to emulsion. Thus the Ilford *L 4* emulsion, when developed with *Microdol* (Kodak) displays no fading after 2 months' storage in dry air at room temperature; yet the Kodak emulsion *NTE* under the same conditions is said by Salpeter and Bachmann [391] to show a 60% drop on developing in *Dektol*. Bachmann and Salpeter [22] prevent fading by vapourising an intermediate layer of carbon on to the section and then coating the preparation with photographic emulsion. Exposure in an inert gas, such as helium, is stated to have the same influence. Both Herz [194] and Ray and Stevens [359] employed this artifice in stripping film autoradiography. They exposed in a carbon dioxide or nitrogen atmosphere.

Whereas exposure in an oxygen-free atmosphere seems chemically reasonable, the restricting influence of carbon vapour deposition on fading cannot be explained. The fading of the *NTE* emulsion, mentioned above, has perhaps other origins. It could, for instance, have arisen through negative chemography, i.e., as a result of oxidation of latent silver nucleates, through contact with the preparation under investigation. In any case, as far as we know, fading phenomena of the magnitude mentioned above under otherwise comparable conditions have not been described so far.

In this connection we should like to oppose the widely held opinion that the preparation must be covered with a carbon layer in electron-microscope autoradiography. According to our own experience with ultra-thin sections embedded in *Epon* or *methacrylate* and with pure *methacrylate* preparations, carbon vapourisation is not necessary. It is a complication which reduces the number of usable preparations as a result of new sources of error. Chemography did not occur with our preparations. In our opinion, this would be the sole justification for carbon vaporisation. Several firms, e. g. *Balzers* of Liechtenstein, offer smaller-sized, easily handled equipment for this. It is suitable also for coating with very thin silica or metal films through evaporation in high vacuum and can be used to prepare impressions of preparations and for various other purposes in electron microscopy.

Recent investigations, expressly concerning autoradiographic exposure of electron-microscope preparations, indicate that exposure *in vacuo* is desirable. This excludes atmospheric oxidation and furnishes definite and reproducible storage conditions under which growth of background during periods up to 2 months is practically negligible with the emulsions most generally used [136].

Weighty problems arise in the interpretation of electron-microscope autoradiograms as a result of the existence of background. Curiously, this circumstance and its consequences are scarcely reflected in the literature. Quantitative data on the magnitude of the background encountered with inactive control preparations are found only sporadically [488]. CARO estimates that the Ilford *L4* emulsion has about 1 silver grain per 30 μ^2. This means over 3 million grains per cm^2! SALPETER and BACHMANN [391] estimate less than 1 grain per 50 μ^2 for the Kodak *NTE* emulsion. FISCHER and WERNER always found background of the order of 10^7 silver grains per cm^2 for the Agfa-Gevaert emulsion *NUC 3.07* [136]; the value was nearly independent of the developer used.

At the present time, the size of the background of most emulsions impedes wider application of the autoradiographic method in electron microscopy. This is not dispelled by the fact that, in numerous publications, reproduction of diagrams with a silver grain density of the order of magnitude of the background creates the impression that there is no background at all to be considered. *One cannot thus warn enough against uncritical interpretation of such autoradiograms.* A rough calculation, based on the activity in the ultra-thin section, its geometrical surface and the exposure, is often enough to estimate the maximum number of silver grains which could be present and thereby to show that the particular "autoradiogram" is merely a random product.

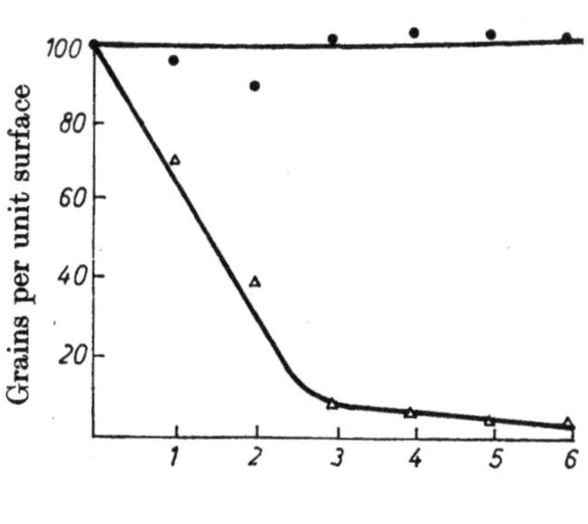

Fig. 78. Background eradication through pre-exposure of emulsion-coated preparations to a H_2O_2 atmosphere, according to CARO [78]. The background (△) was determined through the number of silver grains per unit surface and is referred in each case to the value before treatment with H_2O_2. Practically constant is the number of silver grains present over each *E. coli* preparation, uniformly labelled with ^{3}H-leucine, which are not in the background (.)

Although the desire to reduce the size of background is as vital as ever, no procedure has so far been found which reduces the initially present background through a sort of "artificial fading" without affecting adversely the sensitivity of the emulsion to radiation. Before beginning the real exposure, CARO [78; 82] subjects the ready, emulsion-coated preparations for about 5 to 6 hours to the atmosphere formed above 30% aqueous hydrogen peroxide (*Perhydrol*); in this way the background is lowered to about one-twentieth of its original value. Presumably the number of latently exposed crystals declines without fear of any marked loss in radiation-sensitivity of the remaining emulsion (Fig. 78). The method, also known as "background eradication," was used originally with the *K5* Ilford emulsion. It should really be applicable to other emulsions too. We have, however, not obtained satisfactory results with the Agfa-Gevaert emulsion *NUC 3.07*. It must be noted, incidentally, that there is a potential danger of substance displacement in the preparation through action of the hydrogen peroxide; for example, lipids fixed with osmium are attacked by hydrogen peroxide*.
Recent investigation** has shown that certain metal grids (especially copper) increase the level of background. By using silver grids it has been possible to reduce this background to a minimum.

6.7. Photographic development of very thin emulsion layers

It is not essential to adhere firmly to the instructions given in Chapter 6.4, for development in connection with pretreatment of emulsions or preparation of thin layers. Any photographic developer can be used in principle for monolayers. Where possible, however, one will use the developer suggested by the manufacturer of the emulsion. These are so-called fine-grain developers, regarding the use and crystal size of the emulsions. The time of development must be as short as possible. Over-development is always detrimental—not only with fine-grained emulsions. It modifies the relation of autoradiographically yielded silver grains to background in favour of the latter. Evaluation is thus at least made more difficult. The temperature of the developing bath can be chosen as desired. It ought not to exceed +20° C since the film is thin; the development process would then be too vigorous, bringing a risk of over-development. CARO and co-workers [82] give "development curves" for some emulsions which portray the situation lucidly. According to these, only a small increase in background occurs in the first period of development, whereas latently exposed crystals rapidly undergo photographic development (Figs 79, 80). The end of development time is chosen as the point where development has largely or wholly taken place and the background has still not significantly increased. With some combinations of emulsion and developer, the desired development

* BAKER, J. R.: Cytological Technique, 4th Edition, Methuen, London 1960.
** FISCHER, H. A., H. KORR and G. WERNER: Naturwissenschaften **57** (1970) 450.

has already been attained before the jump in background value. The optimum time of development then lies in the middle of the plateau; in Fig. 79, at about 4 to 5 minutes. It is more difficult when the steep increase in background begins before development of the autoradiogram is complete; this applies, for instance, to the Ilford *K5* emulsion (Fig. 80). Systems of this sort are unsuitable for reproducible work and, especially for quantitative autoradiography, cannot be considered. Development and the following operations are best conducted in suitably sized plastic dishes, glass beakers or the staining dishes known from

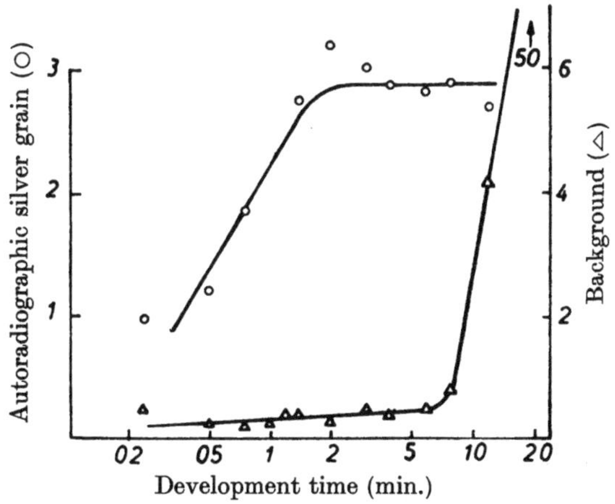

Fig. 79. Development curve for the Ilford *L4* emulsion in *D19* developer at 20° C; from CARO and VAN TUBERGEN [82]. The "autoradiographic" silver grains are denoted with ○, the background grains with △

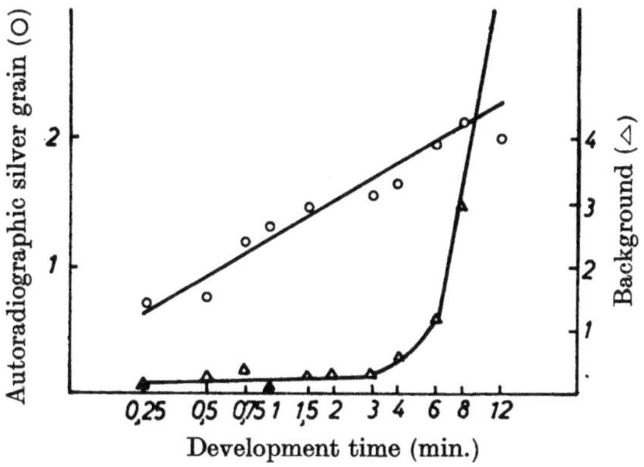

Fig. 80. Development curve for the Ilford *K5* emulsion in *D19* developer at 20° C; from CARO and VAN TUBERGEN [82]. The "autoradiographic" silver grains are denoted by ○, the background grains with △

histological staining technique. The specimen grids are then mounted on glass slides to which they are fastened on both sides with adhesive tape [186; 363; 354], rubber solution [76] or otherwise; or small stands are used, with the help of which the grids are immersed in the bath. Some authors prefer to treat each grid separately with a drop of developer solution [226]. The grid is subsequently placed in 0.5 ml of distilled water in a beaker and the whole dipped into the fixing bath and, later, into water. In this way, the specimens do not break through any liquid surfaces, thus avoiding any damage to the preparation which could possibly result from this.

There is a formal distinction between "*chemical*" and "*physical*" developers. The last-named really first returned into fashion in connection with electron-microscopy autoradiography, after having been scarcely used in photography for decades. They yield appreciably smaller silver grains than do chemical developers since they dissolve a large part of the crystal body. *Physical development* involves precipitation of metallic silver from metastable solutions of reducing agents and silver ions; this occurs predominantly on preformed silver nucleates, yielded through irradiation and which function catalytically. *Physical developers* tend to form a photographic layer of dirty appearance, through which the contours of the adjacent preparation appear indistinctly. It is often hard to recognise silver grains microscopically as such. The reproducibility of the photographic development is not ensured. The prototype physical developer contains 1.1 g p-phenylenediamine and 12.6 g anhydrous Na_2SO_3 in 100 ml aqueous solution. It is used for 1 minute at 25° C to develop thin emulsion layers [21]. The silver grain size lies between 400 and 700 Å — a distinguishing advantage over that from normal chemical development which is about 5 to 10 times larger, depending on the manufacture of the emulsion and the conditions under which the developer acts.

Chemical developers attack the silver halide grain so that a thread-like, often extended and irregularly shaped silver filament or bundle is formed (Fig. 81a). It is a widely disseminated error to assume that the quality of autoradiographic resolution depends on the size of this bundle — that a small bundle necessarily means better resolution. The size of the bundle depends on the time of development, temperature and the developer employed. Developers of this type which are often

➔

Fig. 81. Comparison between usual chemical (a) and compact (b) development. From LETTRÉ and PAWELETZ [260]

a) Nucleus of a chicken fibroblast, labelled with ^3H-thymidine. Contrast improved with lead according to REYNOLDS; developed for 1 min at 20° C in an amidol-containing developer;

b) Nucleus of a HeLa cell, labelled with ^3H-thymidine. Contrast improved with lead according to REYNOLDS; compact development for 1 min at 18° C

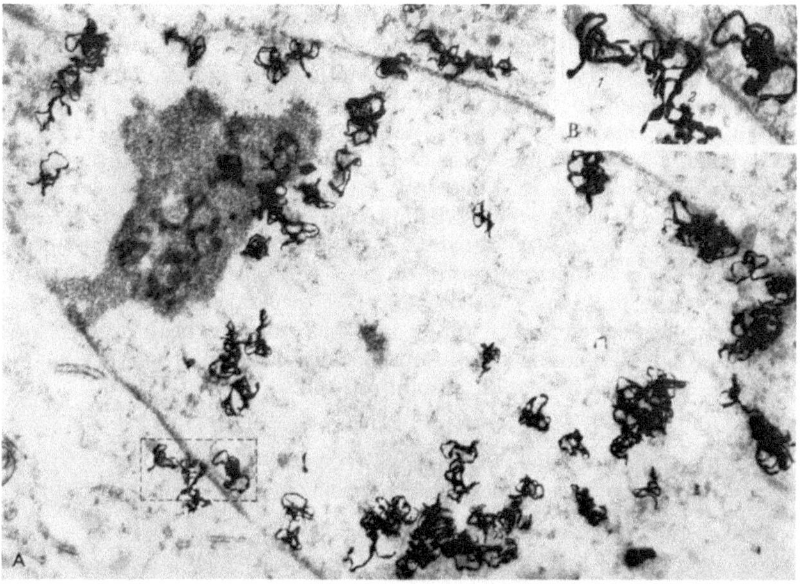

a)

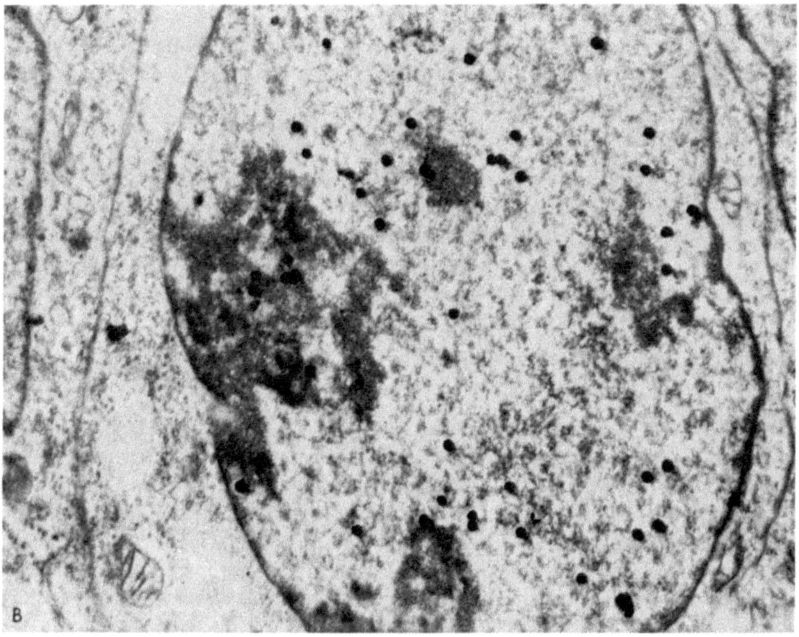

b)

used are: *Dektol* (Kodak); *Microdol X*; Kodak *170*; Kodak *D 19*; and Kodak *D 19* with 0.012% added Kodak *Anti-Fog No. 1* (benzotriazole). Haase and Jung [176] have produced another type of developer, termed *compact developer* to distinguish it from those mentioned previously. Photographic emulsions treated with it yield single, compact silver crystals of nearly circular cross-section. Its principal advantage over previous developers is that electron micrographs with compact silver grains remain distinct when labelling is intense; in contrast, thread-like formations can hide greater areas of the underlying structure (Fig. 81 b). It is sometimes assumed that the position of the primary grain, i. e., the previously latent "exposed" crystal, is identical to that of the finished silver grain [260]; this has not yet been proved (see also Fig. 57 in this connection). Compact development probably has no influence on autoradiographic resolution.

Table 12

Compact development of monolayers according to Haase and Jung [260]

1. Developer:	15.0 g ascorbic acid 2.5 g phenidone 6.0 g potassium bromide 13.0 g potassium carbonate 200.0 g sodium sulphite* 30.0 g potassium thiocyanate These are dissolved in this order in 750 ml of distilled water and the volume made up to 1 litre with distilled water; developing time = 1 minute.
2. Interrupter:	2% acetic acid, for 30 seconds
3. Fixing bath:	Normal negative fixing bath: 200.0 g sodium thiosulphate 20.0 g potassium metabisulphite These are dissolved in succession in 750 ml of distilled water and the volume made up to 1 litre with distilled water. Duration of fixing = 5 minutes
4. Washing:	5 to 10 minutes in gently flowing distilled water.

Small, if not compact, grains are obtained through using so-called *gold-latensification* or gold impregnation, introduced into autoradiography by Salpeter and Bachmann. This technique utilises the action of particular combinations of materials as local elements, a phenomenon known for a long time in electrochemistry in connection with corrosion. Its application of photoemulsions is described here: After autoradiographic exposure, the emulsion film, not yet developed, is treated in

---

* can be omitted.

the dark with an aqueous solution of gold (III) chloride. Traces of gold separate out on to the halide crystals. As a result of a local element action, the gold effects a more rapid solution of the crystals in the developer bath and smaller silver grains are consequently yielded. A 2% aqueous stock solution of gold chloride ($AuCl_3 \cdot HCl \cdot 3\,H_2O$) is used for gold latensification. Shortly before anticipated use, 9.5 ml water are added to 0.5 ml of this solution, 0.125 g potassium thiocyanate is added, then 0.15 g potassium bromide and the final solution is made up to 250 ml with distilled water. This gold thiocyanate solution is unstable and can be used for only one day. The undeveloped autoradiograms are briefly washed and then treated for 30 seconds with the gold thiocyanate solution, again washed and finally developed photographically. SALPETER and BACHMANN use the developer in Table 13.

Table 13

Developer according to SALPETER and BACHMANN [391]

p-Methylaminophenol sulphate (*Methol, Metol*)	0.45 g
Ascorbic acid	3.0 g
Borax	5.0 g
Potassium bromide	1.0 g
made up to 1 litre with water.	

This developer is unstable and should be used for an 8-minute period within 5 to 48 hours after preparation. The grain size of the silver product is then about 500 Å for Kodak *NTE* emulsion; when developed in *Dektol* (diluted 1:2, 2 minutes at 24° C) without gold latensification, this emulsion yields a silver grain diameter of 1200 Å. Gold latensification is stated to increase the sensitivity to radiation of the emulsion to four times that with normal development in *Dektol.* About 3 electrons reaching the layer correspond to each silver grain. It is doubtful, however, if a genuine increase of sensitivity occurs here. This type of development of fine grain yields distinct accumulations of 2 to 3, sometimes even 4, silver grains which always lie within a narrow radius and presumably originate from one single latently exposed crystal. One could contest the assumption of an increase in autoradiographic resolution as a result of this.

The latensification procedure can be used also in combination with other emulsions and developers. Dilution, time of reaction and temperature of the gold thiocyanate solution must be adjusted correspondingly. It must be doubtful whether it is really worth the time involved to obtain debatable advantages. In the end, it is probably only a matter of effects, which, from an objective point of view, do not primarily improve quality and information content of an autoradiogram.

6.8. Labelling possibilities

Many attempts were made early to couple the autoradiographic method with electron microscopy, using also isotopes which, as shown by subsequent experience, are little suitable for this purpose; this was apparently due to inadequate knowledge about the relation between radiation energy and range of the radiation in photographic emulsions. The spectrum of isotopes employed is thus broad, as in light-microscope autoradiography.

Thus LIQUIER-MILWARD [271] worked with ^{60}Co; O'BRIEN and GEORGE [325] with ^{210}Po; MAUNSBACH and ULLBERG [297] with ^{125}I; PELC, COOMBES and BUDD [347] with ^{35}S; GHIARA [155] with ^{14}C; CARO and SCHNOES [81] with ^{32}P; and LUPULESCO and PETROVICI [277; 278] even with ^{131}I.

Up to now there have been no experimental investigations on which emitters are suitable for electron-microscope autoradiography, or on what connection is to be expected in practice between radiation energy on the one hand and grain yield and resolution on the other. As far as possible, therefore, the isotope of lowest radiation energy should be preferred, as follows from the energy loss-route relation (see Chapter 6.2.2.). An idea of the order of magnitude of the maximum radiation range within fine-grained photographic emulsions is obtained from Table 14 for some isotopes often used in histochemistry.

Table 14

Maximum ranges of radiation in fine-grained emulsions

E_{max} (MeV)		Range (μ)	Literature
^{3}H	0.0186	ca 2	CARO and SCHNOES [81]
^{14}C	0.158	90—100	HARBERS (see Section 9.2)
^{35}S	0.167	90—100	HARBERS (see Section 9.2)
^{32}P	1.72	ca 2,000	CARO and SCHNOES [81]

Tritium is the isotope with the weakest known β-radiation. It fulfils best the requirements of electron-microscope autoradiography as far as range and radiation energy are concerned. VAN TUBERGEN [446] was the first to introduce it here and to draw attention to the unique advantages of this low-energy emitter. This was 5 years after LIQUIER-MILWARD's experiments. Tritium has subsequently proved itself satisfactory in high resolution autoradiography and represents probably the only acceptable isotope. During recent years, almost only work with tritium-labelled material has been published although MORICARD and GOTHIE [311] have referred to the usefulness of ^{35}S and CARO and SCHNOES [81] to that of ^{32}P.

We have already mentioned elsewhere that the effective activity of the individual thin-section preparation is generally not particularly high. This has some harmful consequences for the quality of the autoradiograms, such as long times of exposure and high background. This will bring about little difference in most cases, especially investigations on biological material, to which anyhow only a limited amount of radioactive substance can be applied; non-physiological circumstances would otherwise be created. A greater amount of activity may perhaps be introduced by raising the specific activity of the substance concerned. Such substances of suitably high specific activity are unfortunately not always available.

Another way of attaining high activities is to treat the thin layer afterwards with a radioactive substance, i. e., impregnation. By utilising differences in affinity of the intracellular substances to the introduced substance, it is possible to obtain various labelling patterns and even selective labelling of single cell constituents. HOLT and HICKS [201] drew attention to this. GEUSKENS and FICQ [154] "stained" ultrathin sections of *Triturus* ovaries with ^{3}H-actinomycin D. Actinomycin D is an antibiotic which acts cytostatically and probably inhibits RNA-synthesis through irreversible complex-formation with its matrix [120]. An especial affinity to cytoplasm could be demonstrated autoradiographically [154; 94].

FUJITA* has incidentally already pointed out that increased background occurs in electron-microscope autoradiograms of preparations with improved contrast through uranyl acetate treatment; it is due to the natural radioactivity of the uranium.

New methods in cytochemistry could develop through impregnation with radioactive reagents and subsequent autoradiographic localisation of the reaction products.

6.9. Applications and results of electron-microscope autoradiography

Since autoradiography of electron-microscope specimens is still burdened with many difficulties of method, most articles on the subject are of predominantly methodological character. Tritiated thymidine has proved to be a very good test substance in experiments for establishing if a method is reliable and yields genuine "autoradiographic silver grains." Thymidine is a pyrimidine derivative linked to deoxyribose (Fig. 83a). As a nucleoside, it is a starting material in DNA-synthesis and in connection with mitosis is predominantly incorporated into cell nuclei.

* FUJITA, S.: Application of Light and Electron Microscopic Autoradiography to the Study of Cytogenesis of the Forebrain. In: R. HASSLER and H. STEPHAN: Evolution of the Forebrain (Phylogenesis and Autogenesis of the Forebrain). Thieme-Verlag, Stuttgart 1966, p. 180).

It has been possible to prove and confirm this in numerous experiments on many biological species. Thus PRZYBYLSKI [354] worked with *Tetrahymena pyriformis*; VAN TUBERGEN [446] with cell cultures of *Escherichia coli*: REVEL and HAY [362] with larvae of *Amblystoma opacum*; GRANBOULAN and co-workers with, for example, cell cultures of monkey kidneys [164] or with the *SV 40*-virus [165]; and HAMPTON and QUASTLER [180] with parts of intestinal epithelial cells. Although these studies were undertaken to some extent with various methods, it seems very probable that the labelled thymidine is incorporated only in electron-tight parts of the nuclear chromatin. The argument about how far incorporation into cytoplasmatic polynucleotides takes place has not yet been resolved. SILK and co-workers [413; 414] found in-

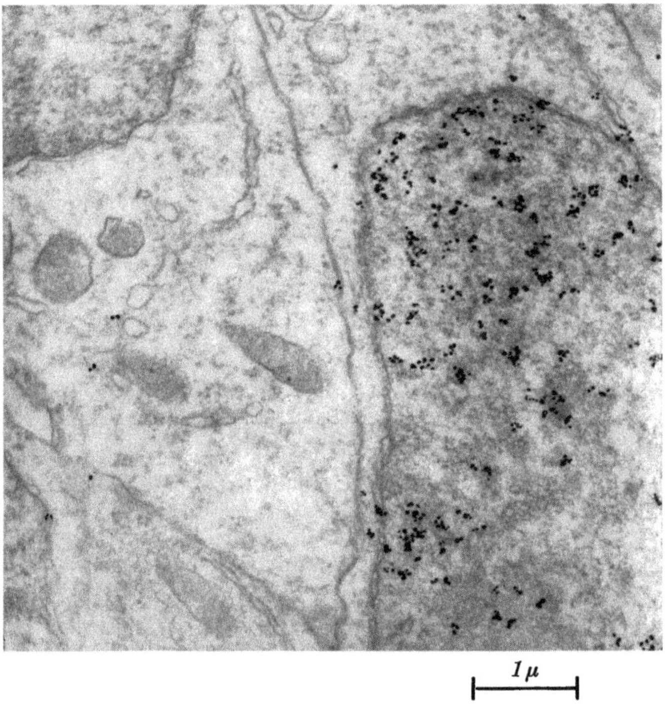

Fig. 82. Electron-microscope autoradiogram of the *Lobus opticus* of a 4-day old chicken embryo which was treated 6 hours before death with 100 μC of ^{3}H-thymidine. Contrast improvement with uranyl acetate. The matrix cell shows strong labelling but the presumed neuroblasts are not labelled.

Method of PRZYBYLSKI [354] and of SALPETER and BACHMANN [391]. *NTE* emulsion. Exposure for 1 month in helium. Gold latensification. Development for 2 minutes at 18° C in *Dektol.*

From FUJITA in R. HASSLER and H. STEPHAN: Evolution of the Forebrain. Thieme-Verlag, Stuttgart 1966, p. 188

corporation in the cytoplasm after longer incubation of cell cultures of monkey kidneys with ^{3}H-thymidine; yet neither MEEK and MOSES [302], KOEHLER and co-workers [235] nor REVAL and HAY [362] were able to confirm this result on other specimens. Possibly the evaluation of further autoradiographic experiments with thymidine will aim at a DNA-differentiation in respect of occurrence and metabolic activity.

Thymidine has thus proved its value not only in cytological studies in light-microscopic autoradiography but also in connection with electron-microscopic technique. Without being able to go into further details, we should like to refer to work of FUJITA and FUJITA [146; 147] and of v. GAUDECKER [151] concerning cell differentiation in the central nervous system (Fig. 82).

RNA-molecules can be detected with the help of labelled uridine (Fig. 83b), a specific unit of ribonucleic acids [134; 224; 87; 361].

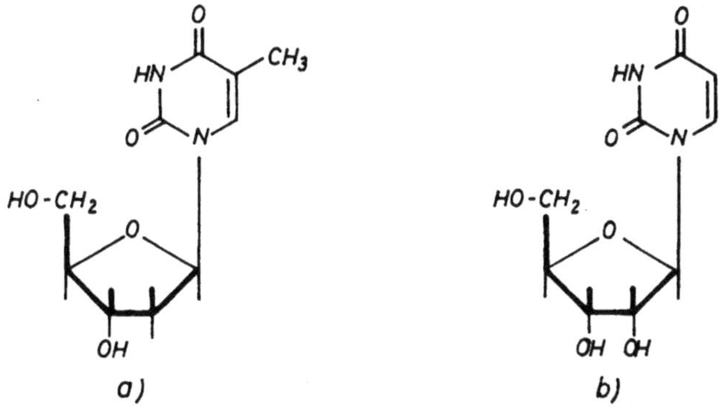

Fig. 83. The nucleosides thymidine (a) and uridine (b) serve for labelling deoxyribonucleic acid (DNA) and ribonucleic acid (RNA), respectively

Through investigations of CARO and PALADE [80] with tritiated leucine it was first possible to obtain morphological proof that the endoplasmatic reticulum is the site of protein synthesis. The newly synthesised proteins are then concentrated over the structures of the Golgi apparatus. Later on, activities can be found in the zymogen granules (Fig. 84). Protein synthesis has been the object also of more recent studies by DROZ and co-workers [111; 109; 110; 113].

CARO and co-workers' results stimulated further work on the process of synthesis and secretion of various glandular cells and also on cartilage metabolism [131; 334; 158; 362]. Some of this work was carried out with ^{35}S-tagged material. The work of ROHR* and co-workers [378; 374; 377; 379; 376] is worth special mention here.

* ROHR, H. P.: Elektronenmikroskopische Autoradiographie. Eine Methode zur Erfassung von intrazellulären Synthesevorgängen. Habilitationsschrift, Freiburg, W. Germany 1966.

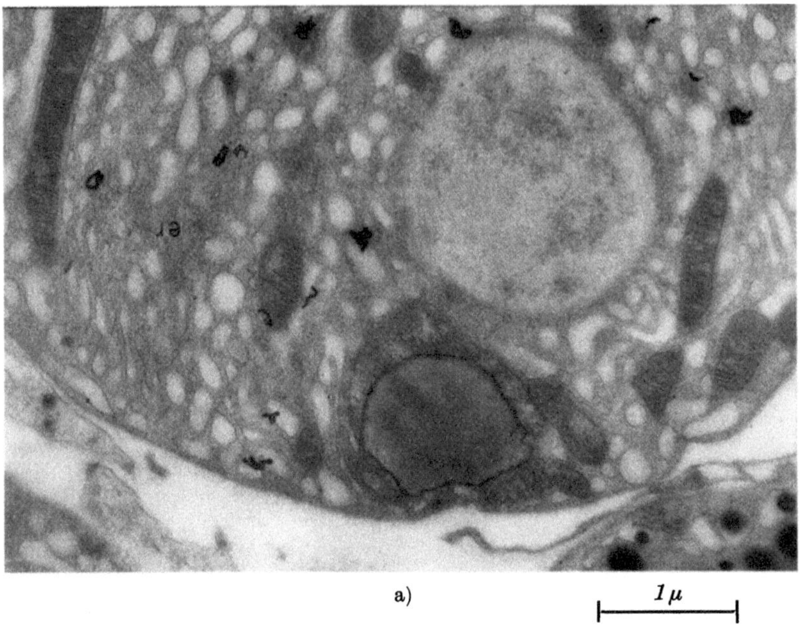

a)

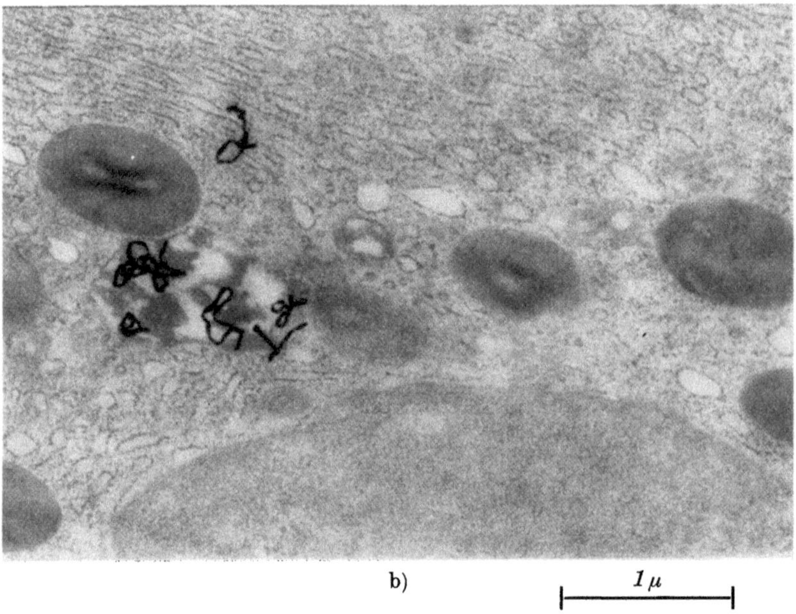

b)

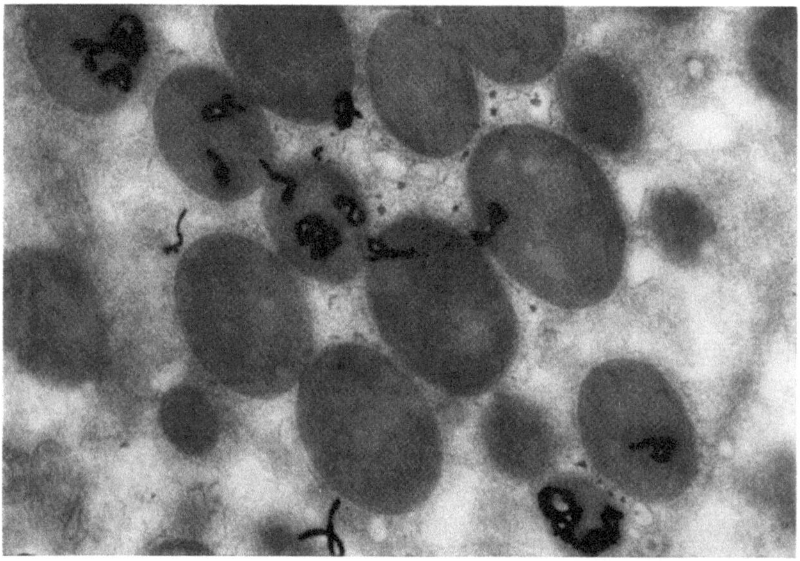

c) 1 μ

Fig. 84. Electron-microscope autoradiograms of CARO and PALADE [80] concerning protein synthesis in exocrinous pancreas cells of guinea pigs, after injection of leucine-4,5-^{3}H

a) Most silver grains are situated above the reticulum 5 minutes after injection;
b) 20 minutes after injection: the activity has been displaced from the endoplasmatic reticulum to the Golgi complex. Most grains are above the condensing vacuoles;
c) 4 hours after injection: the activity is near grown zymogen granules

ROSS and BENDITT [381; 382; 383; 384] studied collagen formation through fibroblasts, taking the example of wound healing.

NAKAI [317] investigated the formation of hair keratin structures, using ^{35}S-labelled cystine. SIMS [415] carried out similar studies with ^{3}H-tyrosine.

Work on the iodine metabolism of the thyroid gland has been done by KAYES, MAUNSBACH and ULLBERG [226]; SHELDON, MCKENZIE and VAN NIMWEGAN [407]; STEIN and GROSS [424; 425]; and others. It is amazing that the isotope used in this work, ^{125}I, is a γ-emitter and yet yielded autoradiograms. If the silver grains are really "autoradiographic," there are two possible explanations of their formation: either a photographically effective release of energy occurs as soon as the radiation enters the emulsion, based on the relatively low γ-energy of 0.035 MeV ("γ-autoradiography"); or secondary processes of energy transfer take place. In the latter case, one would think of the liberation of electrons, the bonding energy of which is very small compared with the energy of a γ-quantum ("*Compton* effect"). The liberated electrons in turn deliver their energy to the photoemulsion. It is, of course, surprising that such a mechanism of exposure can still yield an acceptable autoradiographic resolution at electron-microscopic magnification. A third mechanism to be discussed here might be sought in the so-called internal conversion. This is the simultaneous emission of an electron during *γ-decay*. As far as we know, a conversion coefficient $\frac{e}{\gamma}$ (ratio of converted to non-converted γ-quanta) has not yet been determined for ^{125}I. One may conclude from this that the internal conversion occurs to only a slight extent, if at all.

Another research line is more pharmacologically directed. It is beginning with experiments on intracellular localisation of pharmaceutical and neurochemically active substances. Thus digoxin, a cardiac glycoside, after application as a ^{3}H-containing dose, could be detected in definite ultrastructures of the heart muscle [417; 445]. The site of incorporation of noradrenaline in the adrenic axons, using ^{3}H-noradrenaline, was first determined electron-microscopically by Wolfe, Axelrod and Richardson [485] and Wolfe, Potter, Richardson and Axelrod [486.] The results were confirmed by Aghajanian and Bloom [5] and Budd and Salpeter [71]. Excellent autoradiograms of the storage site of noradrenaline in the central nervous system (Fig. 85) are due to Descarries and Droz [98].

It has been possible with a similar method to demonstrate: the suppression of the cytotoxic action of silicogenic dust particles through polyvinylpyridine N-oxide [144]; the storage of dihydroxyphenylalanine ("Dopa") in the adrenal medulla [121]; and the presence of serotonin in blood platelets [91].

→

Fig. 85. Autoradiograms of rat brain preparations. Injection of a monaminoxidase inhibitor and application of 500 μC of ^{3}H-noradrenaline. Killed 5 minutes after 3-hour injection of the labelling substance into the left lateral ventricle. Histological fixation through perfusion of 3.63% glutaraldehyde in 0.05 M phosphate buffer. Fixation in osmium tetroxide. Embedding in epon. From Descarries and Droz [97]

a) Light-microscopic picture in the region of the *Substantia nigra*. 2 μ section thickness. Emulsion of Ilford *K5* (1 : 1 diluted). Exposed for 1 week. Developed 4 minutes in *D 19* and stained with toluidine blue. Intensely labelled neurons are recognisable. The arrows indicate smaller concentrations of radioactivity in the neuropil with distinct relation to dendrites or nerve endings;
b) Electron-microscope autoradiogram from a part of the *Locus coeruleus*. Thin-section, contrast improved by treatment with uranyl acetate and lead citrate. Carbon vaporisation. Ilford *K4* emulsion (1 :4 diluted). Exposed for 1 month. Developed 3.5 minutes in *Microdol X* at 18° C. A presynaptic nerve ending shows up through especially high enrichment of activity

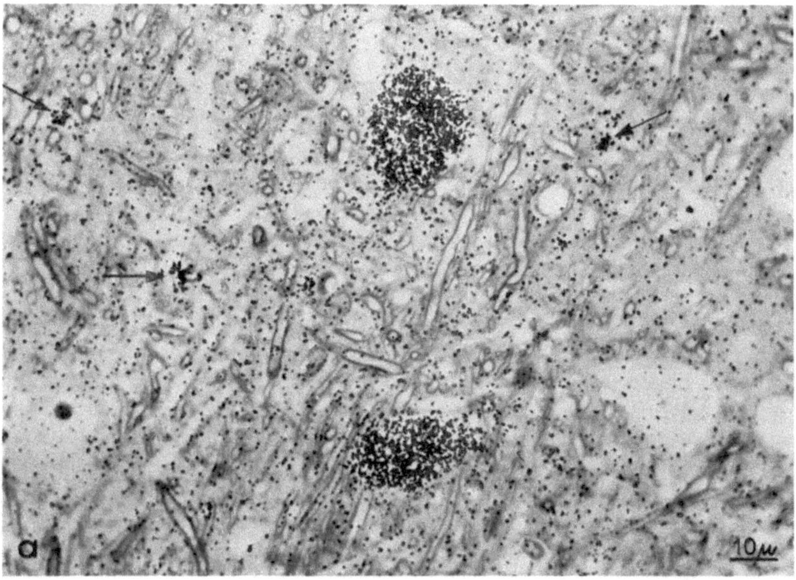
a
10μ

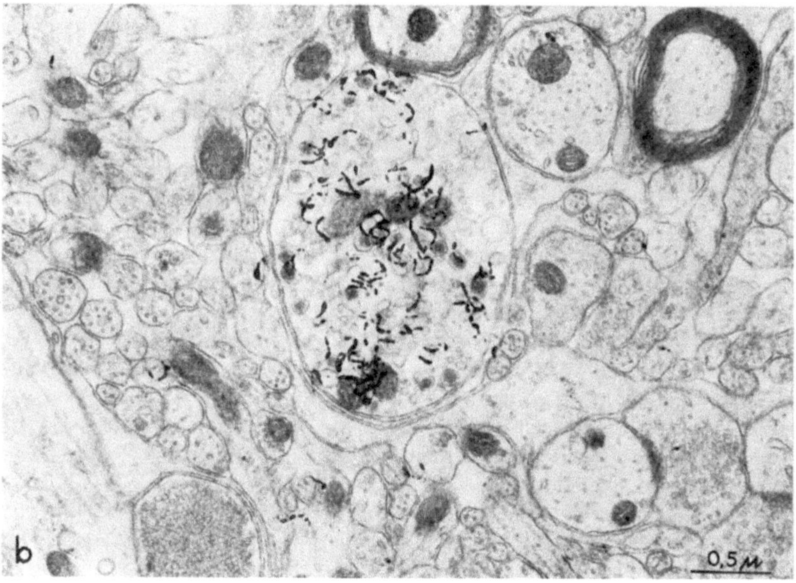
b
0.5μ

7. AUTORADIOGRAPHY AS A QUANTITATIVE METHOD

7.1. Conditions

Under certain conditions, autoradiograms yield a topographical view of the occurrence of radioactive substances and also permit relatively accurate quantitative determinations of the distribution of activity [326; 327; 329].

The number of developable silver halide crystals in a photographic emulsion depends on many factors. These include, to name only a few: the nature of the emitter used; its frequency of occurrence in the studied specimen plane; the extent to which radiation energy is absorbed by the specimen; the sensitivity to radiation of the film material; the duration of autoradiographic exposure; the fading of the latent image; the temperature during exposure. These factors can be divided into those which are variable within certain limits; and those which are more or less automatically pre-determined. Amongst these last named may be counted, for example, geometrical considerations directed by the particular autoradiographic method, such as distance between sensitive layer and specimen or the nature and properties of the photographic emulsion used.

Quantitative autoradiography comprises various procedures for numerically expressing information which can be taken from autoradiograms. This always involves direct or indirect counting of silver grains, referred for comparison purposes to an ultimately arbitrary surface adapted to the particular specimen or to a special aim. The surface to be counted can be chosen in any desired size and its absolute size does not have to be known at all. In microscopic evaluation, for example, a standard surface can be delimited with the aid of a counting screen or diaphragms of any shape. Another way of attaining a definite surface for reference, good for biological specimens, is to choose a surface determined through the nature of the specimen. Suitable would be with protozoa, for instance, the whole cross-section of an individual, visible in the microscope; with metazoa, the largest cell nuclear cross-section.

Since the silver grains in autoradiograms of homogeneously labelled specimens are statistically distributed, it must follow that the average error of a single determination of silver grain density is lower, the larger the surface chosen for counting in the autoradiogram. The reference surface should therefore be as large as the specimen permits. It must never have the order of magnitude of a single silver grain. The number of silver grains per unit surface is called the *silver grain number* or *silver grain density*.

The simplest quantitative evaluation is comparison of the silver grain numbers of various details of the specimen in one and the same autoradiogram. The silver grain density is a function of the radioactivity within the relevant area evaluated. Information is thus obtained about how the occurrence of the particular radioactive substance depends on the topography of the substance. Data can be compared with one another as long as some conditions are fulfilled: The absorption of the radioactive radiation should be constant all over the preparation. The preparation itself must be uniformly thick or extend perpendicularly to the autoradiographed specimen surface to a distance greater than the maximum range of the radiation in the specimen. Finally, both the distance between the surface of the preparation and the photographic layer, and the thickness of the film material must be constant.

Quantitative evaluation of several autoradiograms, where individual comparisons among themselves are wanted, is more demanding. In particular, the autoradiograms must be formed under identical physical and chemical conditions. This is most easily realised when all operations associated with preparation of the autoradiograms are carried out serially, i. e., continuously, or, as far as possible, simultaneously. All preparations must be equally thick — a condition which practically always applies to histological serial layers. Exposure times and details of photographic development, such as temperature and duration of action of the various baths, must be wholly identical.

Quantitative evaluation of autoradiograms derived from different experimental series is possible only when the reproducibility of all decisive preparation conditions is guaranteed. This type of quantitative autoradiography required considerable practical experience and working discipline. Everyone acquainted with autoradiography knows, for example, how variable the fine structure of fully developed silver grains can appear under high magnification, usually for undiscoverable reasons; yet one was of the opinion that, in all these cases, both the composition and the age of the developer corresponded with scrupulous exactness.

Varied times of exposure create no obstacle in principle to the comparison of quantitative evaluations. Correction curves are needed to allow for this, giving the dependence of autoradiographic blackening on the time of exposure (Fig. 89); these must be ascertained experimentally.

7.2 Track counting

If each particle emitted during decay renders developable *more* than *one* silver halide crystal in the photographic layer, characteristic blackening pictures occur. These are made up of single, small, almost

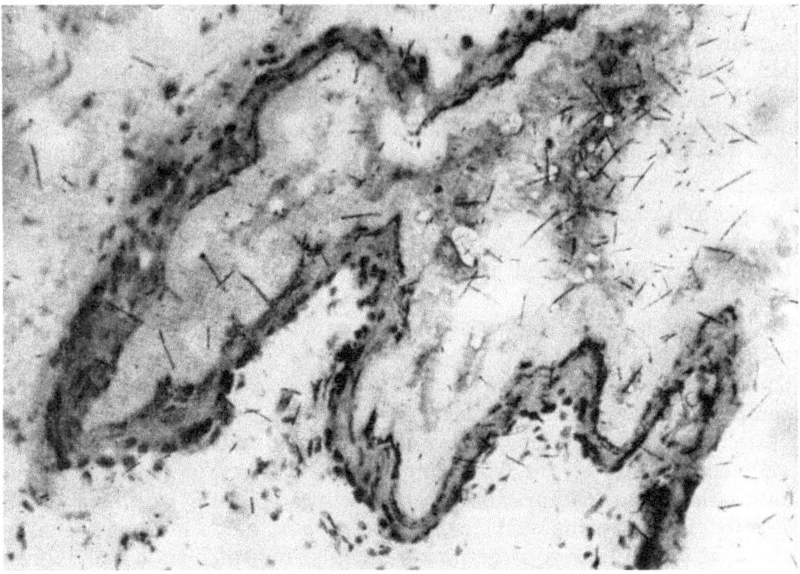

Fig. 86. Stripping autoradiogram of a 5 μ frozen section of the *Tunica mucosa* of the *oesophagus* of a mouse; according to REINHOLZ, BELLOCH-ZIMMERMANN and WIRTH [360]. The tracks originate from ^{210}Po, an α-emitter

linearly arranged series of points which can be fused into nearly uninterrupted lines (Fig. 86). One refers to *track* autoradiograms. BOYD and LEVI [65] were the first to introduce track autoradiography more extensively to biological specimens. It has been subsequently applied often to detect α- and β-emitters as contact-, dipping-, mounting- and also as stripping procedures (Fig. 86) [184; 72; 262; 261; 229; 423; 461; 270; 172]. It is suitable chiefly for emitters with a minimum energy of 100 keV, such as ^{32}P, ^{198}Au, ^{131}I, ^{210}Bi or ^{210}Po. Lower-energy emitters such as ^{14}C or ^{35}S leave mostly irregular, non-linear tracks [171]; their quantitative evaluation is problematic.

In track autoradiography, the blackening of the film material due to radioactive radiation can be distinguished from the single silver grains yielded through other effects; even weakly active preparations, after long exposure, can be evaluated. This is a significant advantage of the method. In addition, extrapolation of the track often permits the origin of the radiation to be localised. Individual radiation sources of high activity reveal themselves as star-shaped blackenings after short exposure time and as a tassel of black spots after longer exposure. DOCKUM and HEALY [101] state that the diameter of a spot is a function of the absolute activity of the associated active particle. According to this, the sum of the diameters of all black spots on an autoradiogram is therefore a function of the total activity of the thin-section preparation concerned; this could be confirmed for ^{106}Ru [101]. The essential quantitative β-track autoradiography dates back to CAMPBELL [72], LEVI [263] and CAMPBELL and PERSON [73]. They were able to show that absolute activity determinations are possible through track counting [264; 265; 266; 267]. The tracks from α-particles are more easily counted than those from β-particles. Every α-particle entering the emulsion leaves a linear track, in contrast to β-tracks. This makes the autoradiographic absolute determination of activity especially easy with α-particles [307; 385; 395; 236]. Most α-emitters are members of the natural decay series of uranium, thorium or actinium. They consequently have radioactive products of decay which in part are likewise α-emitters. In appropriate studies, both the starting element and the α-emitters among the daughter nuclides are therefore detected. By means of track autoradiography it is possible to recognise qualitatively isotopes through the length and shape of the track. Quantitative ratios of the participating radioelements cannot usually be obtained unless the daughter elements behave biologically differently from the original element. Examples of this are known. Thus radium (mass number 224) is taken up preferentially by the skeleton; amongst its daughter elements, ^{212}Pb becomes concentrated particularly in the liver from which it is eliminated as ^{212}Bi after decay [181]. In contrast to silver grain counting (Section 7.3.), quantitative track autoradiography is based largely on visual counting. Counters have been proposed only occasionally, principally to detect heavier particles, such as protons, which have a very short track [32; 422]. Their principle is like that of the counting instruments discussed in the following section.

Nuclear track emulsions are used for recording tracks. They are commercially available on plates and as stacks, without carrier. Liquid emulsions, available in gel form, can be used too. The emulsions *NUC 3.07* and *NUC 7.15* (Agfa-Gevaert) and the Ilford emulsions *L4* and *G5* may be mentioned especially. All larger film manufacturers prepare nuclear track material. If thicker emulsion layers are used, photographic development must be according to the particular temperature cycle instructed by the manufacturer.

7.3. Silver grain counting

The methodological requirements for preparing autoradiograms which can be evaluated by counting individual silver grains correspond to those described in Section 7.1. In contrast to visual track counting, silver grain counting does not differentiate between grains yielded autoradiographically and emulsion background. Only emulsions of very low background may therefore be used; good emulsions should have backgrounds of less than 10 grains/100 μ^2. The background must be determined in control preparations and deducted from the grain density counted each time.

If a visual method has to be adopted, grain counting is unsuitable for extensive routine investigations. The strain associated with counting should not be underestimated, as has been repeatedly pointed out [442; 345; 306]. Errors are moreover possible in direct counting. There has therefore been no shortage of attempts to devise counting aids or to discover measurable entities which are an unambiguous function of the silver grain number. A universally applicable device for grain counting does not yet exist. At the moment it appears hardly possible to construct an automatic counter with a reasonable technical outlay and which can cope with the manifold demands of autoradiographic practice.

Before trying to introduce automatic or even rationalised counting, it should be considered whether this is worth the outlay needed. The decision depends on three factors: the absolute number of silver grains concerned; the amount of material to be evaluated; and the expected duration of the investigations planned. Experience shows that densities up to 40 grains per 100 μ^2 can be counted in the microscope relatively fast and without larger errors by a trained worker. Counting aids are to be recommended for larger counting areas or grain amounts above this value mentioned, especially when much material has to be evaluated [345; 306].

Micou and Goldstein [306] use a projection microscope which permits autoradiograms to be viewed on a frosted glass screen with convenient magnification. The counted silver grains can be marked off on a sheet of transparent paper, using a pen or pencil. This visual counting could be replaced by photometric counting with the help of a so-called Lison photometer [61]. Developments of this sort would appear, however, to have been outmoded by the introduction of microphotometry. One can, of course, count also via the time-consuming detour of using microphotographs; higher grain densities may perhaps be better counted in this way. It is generally worth preparing photographs only in connection with documentation or in standardisation measurements; these are discussed in more detail below.

Other procedures of quantitative evaluation make use of microphotometric measurements [174; 220]. Since the data are obtained electrically, it is only a relatively short step to electronic computer storage [272]. An important difference should be noted between direct visual counting and indirect measurement of grain number. In the latter, the determination is generally not of the accurate number of grains in the relevant area; instead, an effect is quantified which is only indirectly a function of the grain number. Direct visual counting takes in the genuine grain number, independently of the size, cross-section or surface structure of the total grain mass to be counted. Indirect measuring methods cannot distinguish in individual cases whether an object, appearing to the eye as a single grain, is really present as a single grain. It may be evaluated as more than one grain or not registered at all, whichever is by chance shown especially strongly by the particular effect on which the measurement depends. Suitably large amounts of silver grain must be present in order that such errors statistically compensate each other in indirect counting.

There are two basic ways of evaluating autoradiograms microphotometrically: either the reflected light from the autoradiographic silver grains is measured in dark field incident illumination; or transmitted light is used and the diminution in intensity is determined, which is proportional to the sum of all grain diameters. Microscope-photometers, based on the single-beam principle, for evaluation of autoradiograms are manufactured by several firms in the optics trade, e. g. *Zeiss*, Oberkochen, W. Germany; *Leitz*, Wetzlar, W. Germany; *Reichert*, Vienna, Austria [148]. Whether transmitted light/absorption or incident light/reflection is used, depends on the nature of the preparation. If the optical density or absorption of the preparation is comparatively large, or the preparation is optically inhomogeneous, i. e., displays local variations of absorption, then transmission photometry is the wrong choice. *Reflection methods* have been described by various authors [173; 95; 442; 368; 369; 371; 104; 103]. They are suitable chiefly for evaluation of stripping and dipping autoradiograms.

In the reflection method of Dörmer et al [104], incident bright field illumination is used. Since the silver grains, however, cause a very much stronger light reflection than the background, a dark field effect is obtained in which the grains shine on a dark background. The apparatus consists basically of an *Ortholux* microscope (Leitz, Wetzlar, W. Germany) with binocular. An Opak-illuminator for polarisation microscopy is used for the vertical incident illumination. The specimen is delimited through an iris or square diaphragm. This surface is seen in a viewing telescope as a bright spot, its size accurately corresponding to the aperture of the measuring diaphragm. Individual structures of the specimen can be stopped down as desired in this visually controlled way. The essential photometer part with viewing telescope and measuring diaphragm is situated on the binocular. The photometer current is read on a galvanometer, the deflection of which depends linearly on the size of the measuring diaphragm, i. e., is directly proportional to the reflected light. Autoradiographic silver grains reflect light strongly and thus increase the galvanometer deflection, which is a function of the grain number in the area of the specimen delimited by the measuring diaphragm (Fig. 87).

An essential disadvantage of this method is the existence of a reflecting background since background reflection can vary locally, depending on the nature of the specimen. Further, larger errors must

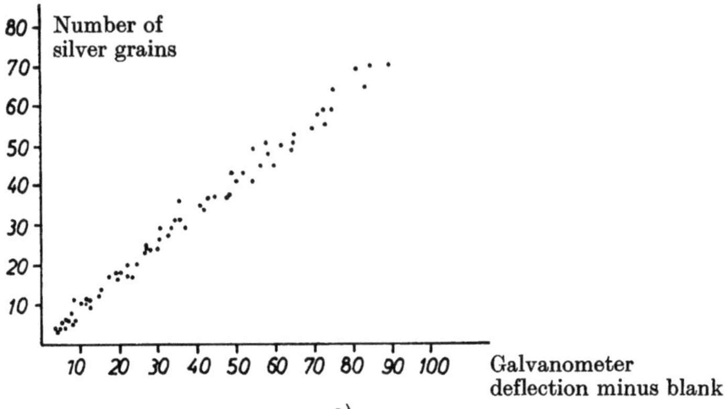

a)

Dependence of the galvanometer deflection on the silver grain number above a labelled myeloblast

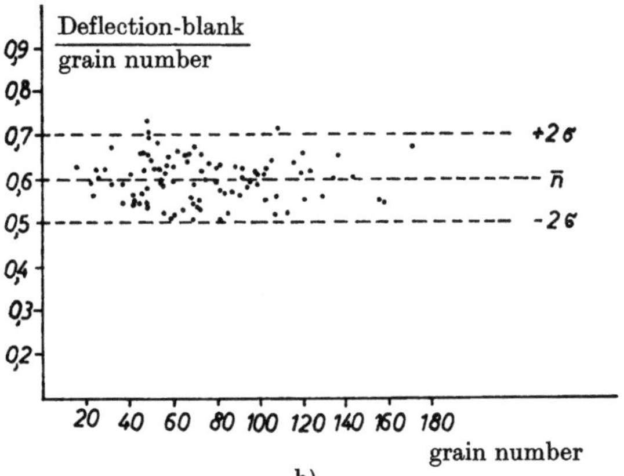

b)

Scattering of photometer values per silver grain above 104 labelled bone marrow cells

Fig. 87. Basic principles of the incident light-reflection microphotometry according to Dörmer et al [104]

be reckoned with wherever, for example, radioactively labelled cells are situated so close to one another that the radii of their scattered light rays overlap, or where smaller groups of silver grains have to be evaluated separately within larger groups [104]. Nevertheless, the incident light reflection method, when critically employed, is superior to any visual counting and is often used. The reason for the widespread use of incident light reflection methods is to be sought less in their perfection than in the nature and type of all those autoradiograms where photographic layer and radioactive preparation are in firm, inseparable contact, even after completing exposure and photographic development. This contact impedes application of other automatic counting devices, just as it may exclude or at least seriously disturb histological, microchemical and photometric studies of the associated preparation. As in the contact method, these disadvantages do not arise when autoradiogram and preparation are treated after complete separation when exposure has been carried out. Evaluation in transmitted light is then possible in quantitative autoradiography.

Absorption methods for determining the silver grain number or analogous entities in autoradiograms have been also known for a long time. As long ago as 1953, DUDLEY and PELC [115] described a device in which a light beam of constant brightness is sent through the autoradiogram. The beam scans extremely fast the preparation surface, the grain number of which is to be estimated. The beam is produced with a cathode-ray tube with electronically driven horizontal and vertical movement, similar to the tubes known from television technique. It is then projected via an ocular down through the microscope on to the condenser. The condenser is combined with a photomultiplier at the exit of which there is a single-channel differential-amplitude discriminator. When the intensity of the scanning beam falling on the multiplier is reduced by 50% or more, or the light beam is interrupted for a brief moment, an electric pulse is yielded which is automatically counted. This technique offers many advantages over numerous other known counting devices; the autoradiogram is digitally evaluated through the discriminator; fluctuating absorption of the background, provided that it does not exceed 50%, does not necessarily prove to be a source of error or otherwise interfere. Stripping- or dipping preparations can also be evaluated. Errors can arise only from the shape and size of individual silver grains. Thus, for instance, U-shaped silver filaments could be counted twice if the beam is twice interrupted while traversing the specimen. The duration of interruption of the beam, however, enters into the result; abnormally large grains are thus more often counted than corresponds to their occurrence in reality. A single determination lasts only a very short time. The whole field of vision in the microscope, $50 \times 50\,\mu^2$, is counted in 0.02 sec. The lower limit is 2 grains per $100\,\mu^2$. Since a fairly considerable outlay of electronic material is necessary, other less complicated procedures have been proposed.

In order to compare silver grain densities along small rectangular sections of stripping film, MAZIA, PLAUT and ELLIS [300] first prepared an enlarged photographic copy of the particular zone on extremely high-contrast film. The photographed autoradiogram is covered with immersion oil and a cover-glass to obtain pictures free of background. One focusses accurately on the plane of the silver grains. A new copy is made from this picture (Fig. 88a), with the help of a camera having a cylindrical lens. It shows more or less thick bands, corresponding to the original autoradiographic grains distribution and frequency of occurrence (Fig. 88b). This band spectrum is evaluated photometrically (Fig. 88c). The procedure can be somewhat simplified by evaluating photometrically without intermediate use of the camera (Fig. 88a). The authors did not consider direct microphotometry to be possible for technical reasons at that time and also with regard to the strongly light-absorbing preparation. Planimetric evaluation of each scanogram area was the essential quantitative operation.

This method of quantitative measurement of silver grain distribution is open to criticism especially where it is concerned with the real distribution of radioactivity in the preparation. In the first place, it appears highly problematic that photographic copies can be obtained which reproduce qualitatively and quantitatively the distribution of blackening of the original. Further, it is very likely that, in areas of high grain density, more than one silver grain is represented by a single line; this means that the translation of the two-dimensional grain distribution into a one-dimensional band pattern effects a levelling of

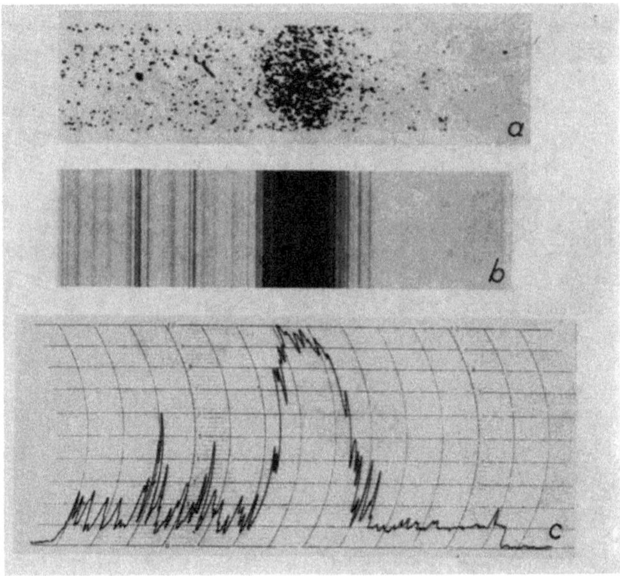

Fig. 88. Quantitative evaluation of stripping-film autoradiograms of strongly light-absorbing preparations. According to Mazia, Plaut and Ellis [300]

a) Microphotograph of the film section to be evaluated;
b) Reproduction of a) through a cylindrical lens;
c) Photometric evaluation of b) in transmitted light

the differences in distribution of blackening. This militates against differentiation of the grain distribution through measurement.
In many cases, the light absorption of the preparation clearly does not hinder quantitative evaluation of the autoradiogram. ALTMAN [7; 8] evaluated de-paraffined dipping-preparations by means of absorption of transmitted light. After subtracting a mean value for the blank absorption of section and emulsion, he found a reproducible linear relation between the grain number within a circular area of 12 μ diameter and the light absorption, expressed as optical density.
KUTZIM [242; 245] proceeded similarly in quantitative whole-body autoradiography. He determined the blackening of organs, denoted by D, as a percentage of those which are the darkest, namely, arterial vessels. D is given by the equation

$$I_x = I_0 \cdot 10^{-D}$$

where I_0 = intensity of light entering the organ
I_x = intensity of light leaving the organ

D is termed the optical density. According to PELC [344], the simple relation,

$$D = 0.4343 \cdot N \cdot a$$

holds between D, N (the number of silver grains present per unit surface of emulsion) and a (the average cross-section of a grain). These equations are valid only if the number of silver grains is relatively low and the grains neither wholly nor partly cover one another. The number of particles emitted in radioactive decay needed to convert a silver halide crystal into a photographically developable state can be determined for a given emulsion. Simple quantitative relations can thus be established between the radioactivity on the surface of the specimen and the data to be determined optically. Equations of this type would, however, apply only in extreme cases, such as low times of exposure or feeble radioactivity, thin preparations and thin emulsion layers.
The range of validity of a simple linear relationship between radioactivity and blackening is relatively small for all radiation-sensitive emulsions. The first action of radiation is to form photographically developable crystals in the part of the emulsion nearest to the preparation. A linear relation can still be expected between blackening of the film and duration of exposure. However, when the parts of the emulsion nearest to the preparation have largely attained the developable state, further increase in the number of developable crystals can be achieved only through radiation components of higher energy. The proportion of these components is comparatively small, in accordance with the energy distribution on the surface of radioactive preparations. A graph of absorption of transmitted light against time of exposure yields a curve climbing from the origin and asymptotically approaching the maximum degree of blackening attainable for the particular film layer (Fig. 89). For the diminishing

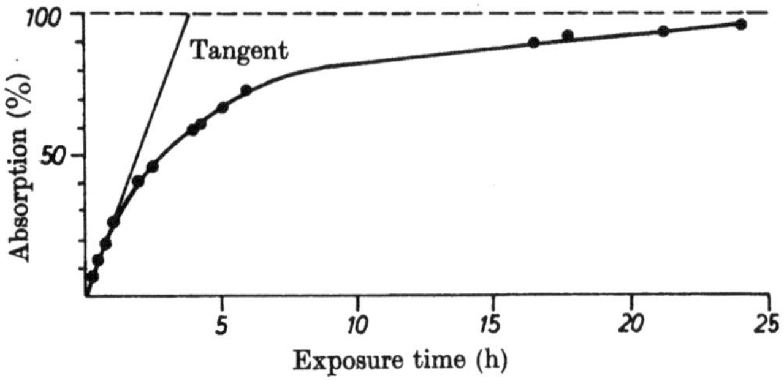

Fig. 89. Increase of blackening with increase in time of exposure. Preparation: tritiated plastic foil with a surface β-emission of -2.28 · 10^6 β-particles/cm^2 · min; emulsion: Ilford *G5*, spread on transparent foil support according to WERNER et al [481]. From FISCHER and WERNER [135]

gradient of such absorption curves there are reasons other than decrease in the number of developable silver grains and consequently also the grain yield.

Grains which do not belong to emulsion layers near the preparation are necessarily more or less optically hidden by other grains already present. As a result, their participation in the absorption of the transmitted light is relatively small and light absorption cannot increase proportionally to the increase in number of silver grains.

The last-mentioned fact shows also that it is not possible to determine activity through silver grain counting on the basis of the usual photometric concentration measurements, according to the LAMBERT-BEER law. This law holds when the degrees of diminution of the transmitted light after having passing through layers of the same thickness are identical and when the total extinction of all layers together equals the sum of their individual extinctions; this does not apply to layers with optically opaque particles. All these quantitative treatments based on the previously quoted formulation of PELC are dubious for the same reason.

DÖRMER [102] termed it "*coincidence*" when several radiation quanta encounter at the same silver grain. Coincidence leads to a varying relation between radioactive decay and the resulting grain number in the sense that increase in grain yield no longer keeps pace with increase in the time of exposure. The curve of the graph would be a straight line if always the same number of radiation quanta led to the formation of one latently exposed crystal. This would be the tangent drawn on Fig. 89. For more accurate evaluation of autoradiograms based on absolute activities, the measured absorption value or the observed grain number must therefore be corrected by projection on the tangent. A measured value of 45%, for instance, would then correspond to a proportionality value of 65%. If one compares the activity of an area, the corresponding autoradiogram of which shows an absorption of 10%, with that of another region of the same autoradiogram with 45% absorption, the true ratio of the activities of the two areas is 10:65 and not 10:45. The proportional value pertaining to a measured value is determined with the help of an absorption curve which is experimentally prepared. A radioactive calibration standard is needed, e. g. for tritium-autoradiography, a tritiated Plexiglas* which can be obtained commercially as a thin plate. It is treated just like a specimen to be autoradiographed, exposed, developed and the absorption of the film material is then measured. This is repeated with various exposure times until the course of the absorption curve and its tangent at the origin is established [135].

This measurement of absorption requires strictest control of the measuring procedure and the guarantee that the measurement is always performed in the same way. The indication of the value must be reproducible for every measured site of every preparation at all times. Manipulation with vague scale divisions or "photometric units" [119] is not enough when their quantitative significance is indefinite or variable (*"semi-quantitative autoradiography"*).

It is easy to carry out standardisation of transmission-photometric measurements with electronic aids. The indicator on the instrument is regulated so that the lightest part of a preparation (e. g., the film material which has not been autoradiographically blackened) yields the full scale deflection, corresponding optically to 0% absorption. The reading at the opposite end of the scale corresponds to total darkness. Such dark regions do not normally occur. Consequently black foil with low reflection is used instead of the preparation, or the aperture of the diaphragm is completely closed. Which is done depends on the particular apparatus. The instrument, if correctly adjusted, now indicates 100% absorption. The dark current of the multiplier is likewise compensated and does not enter into the measurement. Any film blank can be automatically eliminated by setting the absorption at 0% for the autoradiographically unblackened film. The absorptions 0% and 100% are therefore absolute fixed points. They limit an interval within which all measurement values must fall. A higher concentration of radioactive substance in the preparation corresponds to the spot with higher light absorption in the autoradiogram, provided that the absorption of the radioactive radiation by the preparation itself is negligible or constant.

The higher the absorption, the less accurate is the quantitative evaluation. Quantitative autoradiography is out of the question after extremely long exposure or with high local enrichment of activity. Where possible, one should therefore carry out measurements in the sensibly linear initial part of the absorption curve; this facilitates evaluation.

The simple relation, 1% absorption corresponds to a β-emission of $5.2 \cdot 10^6 \beta/cm^2$, is, for example, valid for quantitative autoradiography with

* Polymethyl methacrylate (cf Perspex) (see p. 116).

tritium-containing preparations and Ilford *G5* emulsion, according to the transmitted light method of FISCHER and WERNER [135; 137]. This relation is independent of the exposure time and retains its validity up to 25% light absorption. At absorptions exceeding this amount, the above-mentioned correction procedure, i. e., graphical determination of proportionality values, must be used.

DOMINGUES, SARKO and BALDWIN [107] and MAMUL [285] worked somewhat differently. They determined the activity of the section under investigation by comparison with the blackening of a standard used each time. After the most suitable time of exposure, the autoradiograms of section and of standard were developed under the same conditions and their optical densities were determined. The integral of the optical density curve was plotted against the radioactive disintegrations in the standard. The number of disintegrations of the preparation could be read directly from this plotted curve.

BERLIN and ULLBERG [45] use strip-shaped standards with graduated isotope concentrations. Each standard consists of 14 rectangular shapes of various activities, differing from stage to stage by a factor of 2. They are prepared by dipping photographically developed and fixed X-ray film, serving merely as a carrier, into an aqueous solution of the isotope employed. The radioactivity of the standards is measured in parallel absolute determinations. A standard strip accompanies each preparation being exposed. The activity of organs can be evaluated by comparison with an interpolation of the blackening stages yielded with the standard.

Methods requiring constant use of reference standards, needing preparation and measurement of standard strips, are rather more involved than those based on calibration curves. However, they are less susceptible to errors resulting from random deviations from normal treatment which escape control.

GETSEL [153] describes the preparation of standards for ^{32}P-autoradiography.

7.4. Special features of quantitative tritium-autoradiography

By reason of the low radiation energy, substances labelled with tritium can be detected with such high resolution that intracellular localisation is possible [195; 56; 57; 58]. One can therefore investigate not only material topography but also the kinetics of intracellular metabolism, using suitably labelled material [448; 53; 432]. Investigations concerned with metabolic processes in the cell are in fact amongst the principal applications of quantitative autoradiography today. Some special features of such studies must be noted, arising from the low radiation energy of tritium and the varying densities of the individual cell structures [328].

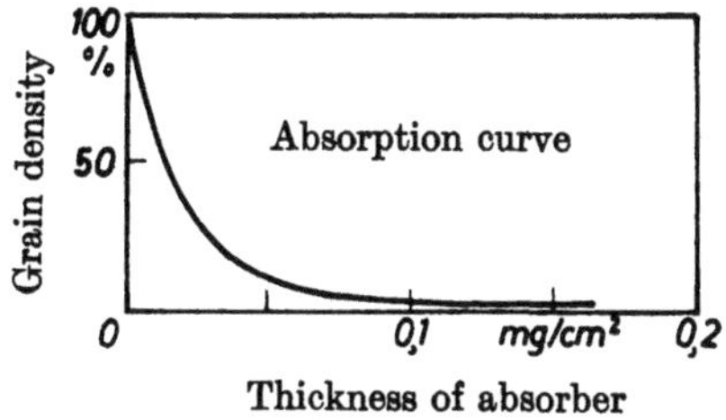

Fig. 90. Dependence of silver grain density on the dry weight of a preparation, according to MAURER and PRIMBSCH [298]

Fig. 90 shows how the silver grain density above a flat ^{3}H-β-source diminishes with increase in density of the inactive absorber layer between radiation source and film. A layer of only 0.05 mg/cm² above the source reduces the grain density to one tenth of its original value. This corresponds to a layer of native tissue, only 0.5 μ thick. This example makes clear the part played by self-absorption in tritium-autoradiography. MAURER and PRIMBSCH [298] were able to show that, for biological specimens also, the mass per unit surface, termed mass density, determines the β-absorption. They determined first the silver grain density as a function of the section thickness for caryoplasm, cytoplasm and nucleolus of mouse liver, after dosage with ^{3}H-tyrosine or ^{3}H-cytidine. If the particular mass densities are chosen as references instead of specimen thicknesses, all three curves coincide within the accuracy of measurement.

A useful concept is the *self-absorption coefficient*. It gives the fraction to which the expected value of silver grain density is reduced through absorption of radiation in the preparation. For a 1 μ liver section, the grains found above nucleolus, cytoplasm and caryoplasm were, respectively, 20%, 60% and 80% of the amounts which would have occurred *without* β-self absorption; the coefficients are thus 0.2, 0.6 and 0.8, respectively. The reciprocal of the self-absorption coefficient is a correction factor with which the measured grain densities are multiplied to

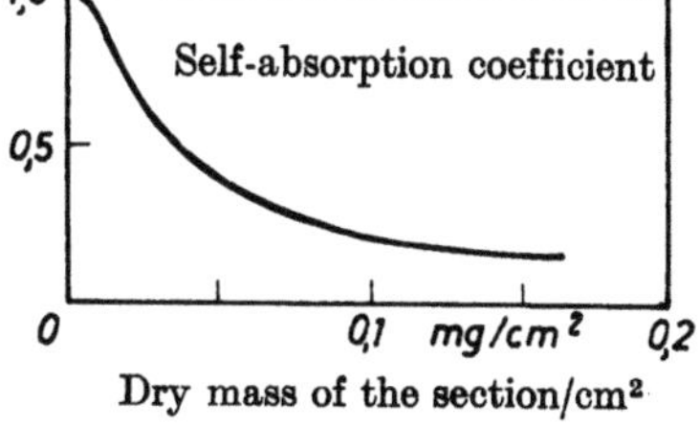

Fig. 91. Relation between self-absorption coefficient and dry weight of the section, according to MAURER and PRIMBSCH [298]

yield grain densities proportional to the activity. In Fig. 91 is seen the variation of self-absorption coefficient with dry weight of the section. The application of such correction factors is necessary in intracellular investigations as a result of the very variable densities [402; 14]. Only with sections up to about 0.1 μ thick is the grain density above the structures studied by MAURER and PRIMBSCH a relative measure for their tritium content (Fig. 92). ^{3}H-autoradiograms of thicker sections can be evaluated when the densities and also the thicknesses of the structures under study are known, so that the real activities can be ascertained. The mass density can be measured by interferometry or radiographically, i. e., with the aid of soft X-ray-, electron- or other radioactive radiation [39; 18].
PERRY [349] treated the mathematical basis for transforming observed silver grain numbers into activity-proportional values. STILLSTRÖM

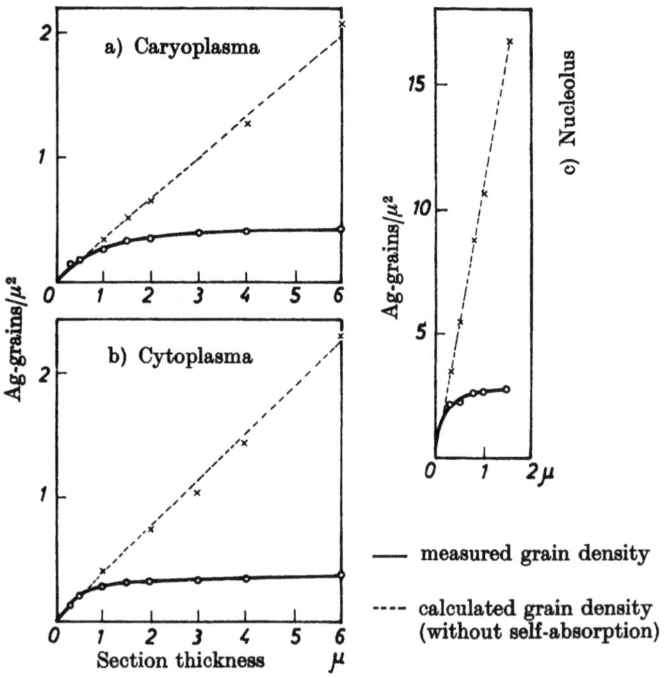

Fig. 92. Silver grain density as a function of section thickness for caryoplasm, cytoplasm and nucleolus

a) and b) mouse liver after dosage of ^{3}H-tyrosine;
c) mouse liver after dosage of ^{3}H-cytidine

Embedded in methylacrylate; stripping film *AR 10* (Kodak). According to MAURER and PRIMBSCH [298]

[428; 429] also studied in detail problems of correction of grain numbers and the influence of background effects, of time of exposure and of variation of cell size on the silver grain number.

Cyto-autoradiographic data can be obtained only on material with a large number of cells, since the labelling in the individual case can deviate markedly from that found in a group of similar cells. This necessarily raises the question of the significance of a result which can be answered with customary statistical methods. It is more difficult when the individual results show scattering which cannot be attributed to insufficiencies of the method. It can be checked in this case if the cells present belong to different populations or types. KASTENBAUM and HANNA [225] developed a statistical model for this, the so-called "Varianzverhältnis-Statistik" or F-test.

As a result of the varied self-absorption of cell constituents, quantitative cyto-autoradiography has become a special subject. We can only intimate its problems. A more detailed presentation of special questions is to be found in the work of MAURER and co-workers especially in SCHULTZE*; they quote extensively literature sources providing excellent access to the autoradiographical studies carried out up to now in the field of cell metabolism.

Quantitative tritium autoradiography is burdened with particular uncertainties resulting from the anisotropic cell density, not only in the subcellular region. Comparisons between silver grain densities above different tissues, e. g. in whole-body autoradiography, demand great caution too. It is quite conceivable here that, where self-absorption of the labelled constituents varies considerably, higher activity is nevertheless associated with inferior blackening. Tritium-labelling should thus be avoided in whole-body autoradiography if there is to be a semi-quantitative estimate of the distribution of a substance.

All other labelling in quantitative autoradiography is above suspicion. In particular, β-absorption is insignificant in ^{14}C-labelling with customary thicknesses of section. This means that blackening of the film is directly proportional to the particular local activity, at least in the early stages of exposure.

7.5. Aids to calculation in work with short-life emitters

The half-life values of the radioactive emitters have not been taken into consideration in the discussions above. This omission is really permissible only when the time of exposure is negligible compared with the half-life. The activity of the preparation then does not noticeably diminish during

---

* See Section 9.2.

its autoradiographic exposure. This applies always to radiocarbon (τ = 5760 years). In principle it would therefore be possible here to prepare several contact autoradiograms from the same preparation which would inevitably be identical, provided that the times of exposure and other preparation conditions were the same. This provides a basis for experimental control. Any differences between expected and observed blackening after repeated autoradiography are a sure indication that not all factors were reproducible during preparation of the autoradiograms. This principle is utilised in histoautoradiography by, for example, co-autoradiographing each time preparations for which the relation of silver grain number and time of exposure is known [30].

In most cases, the radioactive half-life of tritium (12.26 years) can be regarded as large in comparison with the autoradiographic time of exposure; diminution of activity during this time can be disregarded. The situation is, however, otherwise with, for instance, ^{131}I (τ = 8.05 days) and ^{32}P (τ = 14.3 days). In work with these isotopes, two questions must be asked:

1. How long must the exposure be in order to attain the best blackening?

2. How long must the exposure be in a later experiment so that it is based on the same radiation dose (number of radioactive disintegrations) and consequently the same blackening effects are to be expected?

The efficiency of work with short-life isotopes depends substantially on rapid answers to these and similar questions. Various aids can be employed to solve such problems in reasonable time and thus to facilitate work short-life isotopes.

In the simplest case, when the activity of the sample is known at a definite point in time, the time of exposure can be estimated by a graphical procedure of Wainwright, Anderson, Hammer and Lehmann [460]. A nomogram, published by Dumcombe [118], is available especially for experiments with ^{131}I (Fig. 93). It allows the periods of time to be determined during which the same number of disintegrations occur; an example may be given to illustrate its application. Supposing that a preparation, treated with a particular radioactive substance, is autoradiographically exposed exactly 2 days after the (specific) activity of the substance was determined, i. e., 2 days after "zero time." An exposure of 3 days and 4 hours proves to be the most suitable. These two intervals from "zero time" (2 days and 5 [2 + 3] days and 4 hours) on the scales A and C, respectively, are joined on the nomogram and give a reference point on scale B which governs all subesquent autoradiograms. For example, if another autoradiogram is to be prepared 7 days after zero time, the line joining this time on scale A with the reference point on scale B is produced to cut scale C. The last-named then gives the period of time in which the same number of disintegrations occurs as during exposure of the first preparation. The nomogram shows that

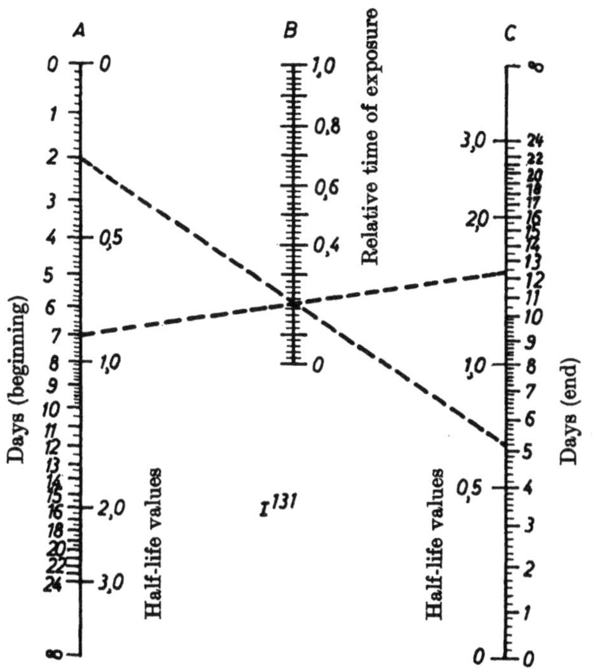

Fig. 93. DUMCOMBE's nomogram [118] for determining the time of exposure of ^{131}I-labelled specimens. Details in text

the time end-point of exposure is after 5.4 days, i. e., 12.4 days after *zero time.*

STOWELL [431] recommends a special slide rule for solving such problems. Each isotope requires its own scale. The iso-dose curves of FLINN [139] are independent of the nature of the isotope and its half-life. Their use demands, however, some experience in handling exponential functions.

7.6. Quantitative autoradiography of electron-microscope preparations

Sporadic contributions to "*quantitative electron-microscope autoradiography*" [69; 20] have been made, despite all the difficulties of method in preparing electron-microscopic autoradiograms (Chapter 6.4.), difficulties which concern above all those factors where reproducibility is a vital condition for quantitative work. Thus ROHR, SEITER and SCHMALBECK* studied conditions and limitations of quantitative autoradio-

* unpublished.

graphy in electron microscopy as applied to kinetic investigations on glandular cells. After detailed discussion of the theoretical and practical requirements they conclude that it is not possible at present to provide with success purely quantitative information on secretion processes; but that semi-quantitative evaluation is nonetheless possible, permitting an estimate of the order of magnitude of the progress with time of synthesis of secretion proteins.

Each of several mice was injected *post partum* with 750 μC leucine-4,5-^{3}H i. p. The mammary glands were cut out at various times between the 5th and 240th minute after injection. Semi-quantitative estimation was done through determining the percent of silver grain distribution above the cell compartments, K_i, of interest. The percent surface of the relevant cell compartments was also determined morphometrically, so that a value could be calculated from the so-called *relative specific localisation*, given by $\frac{\%\ \text{silver grains in}\ K_i}{\%\ \text{surface of}\ K_i}$.

Similar studies were made by Droz and Bergerson [112] and Droz [109; 110] on mitochondrial protein synthesis; and by Salpeter [390] on the distribution of acetylcholinesterase at motor endplates of mouse vertebrate twitch muscles.

One may assume that quantitative evaluation in this field will gain importance as improvements in high resolution autoradiography are made.

7.7. Application and results of quantitative autoradiography

Quantitative autoradiography is carried out on specimens of essentially histological nature. Few applications are known in other domains, except measurements of radiation dosage.

Determination of *dosage* — like the mere detection of radiation with films — is not in itself autoradiography. The blackened image does not represent the distribution of the emitting substance in the sense of a specimen autoradiogram. Measurement of neutron density is a special case. This involves genuine autoradiographic detection of radioactive elements in metal sheets which have been activated by neutrons but where there is no interest in localisation of the emitter itself, however. The activity of detector foils, which is proportional to the neutron density, blackens an adjacent radiation-sensitive emulsion and this can in turn be a measure of the neutron flow [126].

Bhatnager and Ghosh [49] differentiated active and inactive inclusions in polished samples of ore by quantitative autoradiography; this could be of interest in *geological investigations*. The data help characterise the mineralogical composition and can also give information about the history of orgiin of the ore. Quantitative determination of the isotope composition of a mineral may even be possible from the ratio of the number of active and of non-labelled constituents. Similar procedures are used in *metallurgy* for measuring dentritic segregation in steel [273].

Quantitative autoradiography has some importance in *chemical analysis* and in testing purity of radiochemicals. This requires separation of the substances by one- or two-dimensional electrophoresis or chromatography. The details of the method, as far as they concern preparation of autoradiograms, have been discussed in Section 4.2. Quantitative evaluation aims at determining either the absolute activity per spot, or activities based on a reference spot. Autoradiographic activity determination is recommended only for very low activities, e. g. rates of emission of less than 100 impulses per minute per spot. Liquid scintillation counters give more accurate and more quickly obtained results if qualitative autoradiography shows the presence and position of a radioactive spot and the blackening indicates higher activity [418; 419]. Apparatus has been developed especially for thin-layer plates. With these so-called *zonal scrapers*, strips, 1, 2 or 5 mm wide, of the layer can be rapidly and cleanly scraped off and measured in a continuous automatic procedure. This *zonal scanning* is a highly sensitive procedure for detecting tritium also and is even almost as efficient as autoradiographic procedures with regard to resolution in one-dimensional separations [418].

Activities are otherwise determined through photodensitometry of spot blackening. Not only local silver grain densities are of interest; the particular spot size and grain distribution must be considered in order to obtain the total activity per spot. This contrasts with microphotometric evaluation of autoradiograms of light-microscope specimens. The autoradiogram is best scanned and the transmitted light recorded. The light absorption is directly proportional to silver grain density, at least at low blackening, and is therefore directly proportional also to the activity. Apparatus for continuous measurement of the optical density of coloured chromatograms and electropherograms is often used for biological investigations. An auxiliary apparatus, suitable for quantitative autoradiography, is available also for the Eppendorf photometer (Firm of Netheler and Hinz, Hamburg, W. Germany). Evaluation is then carried out by comparing the relevant areas under the recorded curves with one another or with an analogously treated standard spot of the scanned surface. Radebrecht and Binnewies [357] autoradiographically determined ^{32}P-labelled phosphatides, which had been separated by paper chromatography, with the help of a calibration curve, according to which extinction and activity were linearly related.

Another possibility of evaluating paper chromatograms in particular is based on a relation between spot activity, A_0 (μC) and maximum film blackening S_{max} within a chromatogram spot. This relation, due to Narath and Gundlach [319] is:

$$A_0 = \frac{F \cdot d}{t} \cdot 10^{\frac{\log(10^{S_{\max}} - 1) + b}{a}},$$

where F = surface area of the chromatogram spot in cm^2
d = thickness of the paper in cm
t = time of exposure in days.

The values for a and b are derived from calibration measurements and the so-called *linear blackening* relation:

$$S_{\max} = \log(10^{S_{\max}} - 1) = a \cdot \log \frac{A_0 \cdot t}{F \cdot d} - b.$$

Autoradiographic determinations of activity have been made also in connection with WEISZ' [466; 467] *ring oven technique* for separation and microanalytical detection of very small amounts of substance [471; 335; 472; 469]. Here, too, autoradiography may be replaced by liquid scintillation measuring technique; the limit of detection with the latter is still lower than that given by WEISZ and KLOCKOW [470] for semi-quantitative determination of ^{14}C activities in ring oven autoradiography, namely, ca 1 pC.
The technique of automatic variation of exposure time is worth mentioning from the point of view of method. The filter with the ring of material to be evaluated is cut along a radius and pressed against X-ray film so that slipping is impossible. In the course of a slow rotation, the filter is gradually raised from the X-ray film, beginning at the cut edge; this terminates exposure. After development, the autoradiograms thus obtained display a ring with increasing blackening. The active substance where the filter was first raised is only briefly in contact with the film; and that at the other end of the ring is in contact for the whole duration of the rotation ("*Ring-Chronoautoradiography*"). The rotation can be performed discontinuously also and the corresponding autoradiogram is then a ring-shaped staircase optical wedge.
The principle inherent in the method is that at least one sector of the ring will show blackening corresponding to a reference standard. The relevant time of exposure can be determined from the angle turned from the starting point which enables the sought radioactivity to be calculated.
In Section 6.8., we mentioned incubation of histological preparations with radioactive reagents as a qualitative histological method fully comparable with normal staining procedures. Similar reactions are known in cytochemistry, especially in connection with qualitative autoradiographic detection of stored substances [89; 410; 341]. BARNARD and MARBROOK [27] examined the possibility of selective autoradiographic detection of some substances based on their functional groups, using more or less specifically reacting tritium-labelled reagents. They used tritiated acetic anhydride (0.4 M) in pyridine/acetonitrile and acetylated amine, hydroxyl and thiol groups in macromolecules. After a definite reaction

time with the acetylation agent, the number of labelled groups ceases to increase. It may be taken that all groups capable of reaction have indeed reacted. The autoradiogram shows qualitatively the position and distribution of these groups within the cell. Further, it permits the absolute number of labelled functional groups to be determined, when the grain yield is considered; this gives an insight into the spatial constitution of the macromolecules.
Applications of quantitative autoradiographic methods to biological specimens may be classified roughly into the following groups:

a) Investigations of metabolism of bone, cartilage and connective tissue, especially with regard to incorporation of bone-seeking elements (cf chapter 4.3.4.),

b) Studies of general metabolism of substances in healthy or pathologically modified tissue applied orally or by injection [244],

c) Investigations on DNA- and RNA-metabolism, especially concerning mitosis.

Quantitative studies of the metabolism of bone and cartilage were among the first applications of autoradiography and are still based to some extent on the nuclear track method [114; 73; 62; 16; 15; 38; 293; 290; 443; 221]. The first data were obtained about the extent of metabolic processes in bone tissues, the turnover of numerous inorganic ions, and the radiation danger associated with uptake of such elements*.
Vincent, Haumont and Roels [457] worked out a procedure for quantitative microautoradiographic determination of bone phosphorus, based on neutron activation of bone sections.
In connection with group b) above, we should like to refer only to studies of iodine- [316; 170; 322] and sulphur-metabolism [63; 243; 304]. Amongst themes have been measurements of the extent of metabolic activity of endocrine glands. Oehlert** has compiled a comprehensive survey especially devoted to the orthology and pathology of sulphur metabolism in cells.
Work on metabolism in tumours belongs to the third group, of quantitative histoautoradiography [259; 330]. For example, it is possible to estimate the malignancy of a tumour through counting labelled cells. The possibility at present of testing objectively the efficiency of mitotic inhibitors by autoradiography seems more important than the diagnostic aspects of such work [404].
Quantitative autoradiography is especially valuable also in research on mitosis itself. Present knowledge about duration of turnover rate and the phases during division for various types of cell depend largely on investigations with labelled thymidine (Section 6.9.). Of cardinal impor-

---

* cf footnote to page 39.
** See Section 9.2.

tance here is the determination of the DNA-replication time, the so-called S-(synthesis)period. Using autoradiographic experiments with ^{32}P, HOWARD and PELC [204; 205; 206; 207] were the first to conclude that the process of DNA-replication is restricted to a definite part of the interphase. A view of cell growth thus became possible: The DNA-synthesis period (S) follows a postmitotic, pre-synthetic pause (G_1). It is in turn followed by a premitotic pause (G_2), at the conclusion of which the real mitosis begins.

The duration of the S-period of a cell type can be measured on autoradiograms by counting labelled and non-labelled dividing cells as a function of time, following a dose of ^3H-thymidine [355; 336; 233]. A single injection of tagged thymidine suffices to label all cells which are in the S-period at the moment of injection. As time passes, more and more of these labelled cells pass through the G_2-peroid and on through mitosis. If the interval between injection of ^3H-thymidine and killing of the animal is less than G_2, no labelled dividing cells will be observed yet. If this interval exceeds G_2, the first labelled dividing cells appear. If the interval is still larger than $G_2 + M$, all dividing cells are labelled. This is maintained until the duration of the experiment exceeds $G_2 + M + S$. New, non-labelled dividing cells then appear. By counting all labelled states as a function of time after injection, the lengths of the S-period, the $G_2 + M$ period and the G_1-period can be quantitatively determined under certain conditions.

Labelling with *two isotopes* has yielded noteworthy results in quantitative evaluation of autoradiographic experiments. HILSCHER and MAURER [197] introduced this dual labelling into research on mitosis and it has been frequently employed since [350; 257; 258; 351; 196]. We can consider the principle only briefly here. It consists of giving experimental animals a first injection of ^3H-thymidine and, after an interval Δt, a second injection, this time of ^{14}C-thymidine. About 30 minutes after this second injection the animal is killed and autoradiograms are prepared. All cells which are in the S-period at the moment of the first injection are labelled with ^3H as a result. During the interval Δt, some of the ^3H-labelled nuclei pass from the S-period into the G_2-period. At the same time, unlabelled nuclei leave the G_1-period for the S-period. The second injection labels — but this time with ^{14}C — all cells in the S.period at that moment. The autoradiograms then show nuclei with three different types of labelling: 1. Only ^3H-labelled; these have quit the S-period between the first and second injection. 2. Only ^{14}C-labelled; they have appeared in the S-period between the injections. 3. ^3H- and ^{14}C-labelled; these were in the S-period at the time of both injections. In the autoradiogram, the silver grains yielded from ^3H decays can be distinguished from those from ^{14}C decays in that the relatively soft β-radiation from the tritium has a smaller range than the radiation from ^{14}C. Consequently, the tritium-containing nuclei are recorded autoradiographically with higher resolution. In contrast, ^{14}C yields diffusely distributed silver grains.

The fraction of each of these three labelling types can be determined by counting and, under certain conditions, the length of the S-period can be calculated. It is given by the equation below, on the assumption for instance, that the frequency distribution of the nuclei remains constant during a generation cycle ("*steady state*"):

$$\text{Duration of S-period} = \frac{\text{number of } ^{14}\text{C-nuclei (with or without } ^{3}\text{H)}}{\text{number of nuclei labelled only with } ^{3}\text{H}} \cdot \Delta t.$$

An observation made by PILGRIM, LENNARTZ, WEGENER, HOLLWEGE and MAURER [352] on various species is interesting in this connection; diurnal fluctuations in the ^{3}H index and the mitotic index occur. The ^{3}H-index is the ratio of the number of cells labelled with ^{3}H-thymidine to the total number; the mitotic index is the ratio of the number of labelled dividing cells to the total number of dividing cells. These indices show distinct maxima at ca 6 o'clock morning and evening. The variations in ^{3}H-index are interpreted as partial synchronisations of the cell; at certain times of the day, an above-average number of nuclei leaves the G_1-period for the DNA-synthesis period.

These examples may illustrate how autoradiographic methods are useful and indispensable in quantitative studies of DNA- metabolism. Investigation of the magnitude of protein synthesis [254; also Section 9.2] and of nucleic acid and protein metabolisms of the cell, could be ranged along with them. These cannot, however, be discussed here in more detail.

8. APPENDIX

Dates in the historical development

1867 Niepce de St. Victor discovered the blackening of silver chloride and silver bromide through uranium salts and explained this as due to luminescence.

1896 Henri Becquerel showed that photographic emulsions are darkened by uranium salts even when they had not previously been excited with light.

1898 Marie and Pierre Curie proved through their epoch-making isolation of radium sulphate from pitchblende, that various forms of naturally occurring radioactivity exist.

1904 E. S. London prepared the first histoautoradiogram; he exposed a photographic plate to a frog which had inhaled radium emenation.

1924 A. Lacassagne was the first to use autoradiography systematically, to detect incorporation of polonium in biological material.

1933 Tamann and Bandel utilised autoradiography in metallurgy; only few radioelements in the natural decay series were available in concentrated form.

1945 et seq The hectic development of atomic physics assisted a rapid development of autoradiography. Artificial radioisotopes became increasingly available alongside the naturally radioactive nuclides. Many new emulsions, originally developed for detection of radiation and particles in atomic research, were tested for their usefulness in autoradiography.

1946 L. F. Bélanger and C. P. Leblond improved resolution by using liquid, molten emulsions in histoautoradiography.

1950 The stripping film technique found wide application through S. R. Pelc.

1954 J. S. Arnold described autoradiography with nuclear track emulsions. Subsequently H. Levi and C. Levinthal developed their application in β-track autoradiography and in quantitative work.

1956 J. Liquier-Milward made the first experiments in autoradiography of electron-microscopic specimens.

9. BIBLIOGRAPHY

The figures in pointed brackets after each reference refer to the page(s) in the text on which the reference is quoted.

9.1. Cited literature

[1] Ackerman, N. B., A. S. McFee and A. J. Madsen: Increased sensitivity of in vivo radioautographic films. Radiology **84** (1965) 356.

[2] Ackerman, N. B., A. S. McFee and O. H. Wangensteen: Refinements in technique of in vivo radioautography of the stomach. Surgery **51** (1962) 295. —⟨59, 60⟩—.

[3] Ackerman, N. B., D. B. Shahon, A. S. McFee and O. H. Wangensteen: Recognition of gastric cancer by in vivo radioautography. Ann. Surg. **152** (1960) 602. —⟨59, 60⟩—.

[4] Adams, M. D. and R. K. Steunenberg: Some metallurgical applications of autoradiography. Nucl. Sci. Abstr. **16** (1962) Abstr. No. 6684. —⟨10⟩—.

[5] Aghajanian, G. K. and F. E. Bloom: Electron microscopic autoradiography of rat hypothalamus after intraventricular H^3-norepinephrine. Science **153** (1966) 308. —⟨138⟩—.

[6] Albanus, L., L. Hammarström, A. Sundwall, S. Ullberg and B. Vangbo: Distribution and metabolism of H^3-atropine in mice. Acta physiol. scand. **73** (1968) 447. —⟨47⟩—.

[7] Altman, J.: Regional utilization of leucine-tritium by normal rat brain. Microdensitometric evaluation of autoradiograms. J. Histochem. Cytochem. **11** (1963) 741. —⟨149⟩—.

[8] Altman, J.: Differences in the utilization of tritiated leucine by single neurones in normal and exercised rats: An autoradiographic investigation with microdensitometry. Nature **199** (1963) 777. —⟨149⟩—.

[9] Appelgren, L. E., A. Nelson and S. Ullberg: Distribution of Y^{91} in mice studied by whole-body autoradiography. Acta Radiol. (Ther.) Stockholm **4** (1966) 41. —⟨48⟩—.

[10] Appleton, T. C.: Autoradiography of soluble compounds. J. Roy. Micr. Soc. **83** (1964) 277. —⟨78⟩—.

[11] Appleton, T. C.: Resolving power sensitivity and latent image fading of soluble compound autoradiographs. J. Histochem. Cytochem. **14** (1966) 414. —⟨78⟩—.

[12] Appleton, T. C.: Storage of frozen materials for cryostat sectioning and soluble compound autoradiography. J. Roy. Micr. Soc. **87** (1967) 489. —⟨78⟩—.

[13] Appleton, T. C.: Zusammenfassende Übersichten zu den Versuchen der autoradiographischen Darstellung leichtlöslicher Substanzen. Acta Histochem. (Jena) Suppl. VIII (1968) 115. —⟨38, 78, 88⟩—.

[14] Arnold, G.: An autoradiographic study of RNA synthesis in isolated salivary glands of *Drosophila hydei*. I. Autoradiographic studies. J. Morph. **116** (1965) 65. —⟨154⟩—.

[15] Arnold, J. S., W. S. S. Jee and K. Johnson: Observation and quantitative radioautographic studies of Ca^{45} deposited in vivo in forming Haversian system and old bone of rabbit. Amer. J. Anat. **99** (1965) 291. —⟨161⟩—.

[16] Arnold, J. S., K. E. Johnson and W. S. S. Jee: Quantitative radioautographic study of the concentration of in vivo fixed *Ca-45* in new and mature bone. Fed. Proc. **13** (1954) 421. —⟨161⟩—.

[17] ASUNMAA, S. K.: Silver-activated nitrocellulose as recording material for X-ray microscopy. Nature **186** (1960) 1036. —⟨121⟩—.

[18] ATHERTON, D. R. and W. S. S. JEE: Preparation of Sr^{90} standard in plastic block for densitometric evaluation of radioautograms. Nucl. Sci. Abstr. **20** (1966) Abstr. No. 2546. —⟨154⟩—.

[19] AXELROD, D. J.: An improved method for cutting undecalcified bone sections and its application to radioautography. Anat. Rec. **98** (1947) 19. —⟨38⟩—.

[20] BACHMANN, L. and M. M. SALPETER: A quantitative approach to high resolution autoradiography. In: The 3rd European Conf. on Electron Microscopy, Prague 1964, Vol. B. 15. —⟨157⟩—.

[21] BACHMANN, L. and M. M. SALPETER: Zur Autoradiographie im elektronenmikroskopischen Bereich. Naturwissenschaften **51** (1964) 237. —⟨112, 128⟩—.

[22] BACHMANN, L. and M. M. SALPETER: Autoradiography with the electron microscope; a quantitative evaluation. Lab. Invest. **14** (1965) 1041. —⟨92, 94, 112, 124⟩—.

[23] BACHMANN, L. and M. M. SALPETER: Absolute sensitivity of electron microscope radioautography. J. Cell Biol. **33** (1967) 299. —⟨112⟩—.

[24] BÄCKSTRÖM, J., E. HANSSON and S. ULLBERG: Distribution of C^{14}-DDT and C^{14}-Dieldrin in pregnant mice determined by whole-body autoradiography. Toxicol. appl. Pharmacol. **7** (1965) 90. —⟨48⟩—.

[25] BARIGOZZI, F. and P. C. LENSI: The application of radioautographic techniques in metallurgy, and the study of segregations. Met. Ital. **55** (1963) 129. —⟨10⟩—.

[26] BARKER, A. N., H. O. W. RICHARDSON and N. FEATHER: An emission microscope for photoelectron autoradiography. Res. **3** (1950) 431 and Nucl. Sci. Abstr. **4** (1950) Abstr. No. 6034. —⟨119⟩—.

[27] BARNARD, E. A. and J. MARBROOK: Quantitative cytochemistry using directly applied radioactive reagents. Nature **189** (1961) 412. —⟨160⟩—.

[28] BARTELSTONE, H. J.: Radioautography. J. dent. Med. (New York) **20** (1950) 307. —⟨44⟩—.

[29] BARTELSTONE, H. J., J. D. MANDEL, E. OSHRY and S. M. SEIDLIN: Use of radioactive iodine as a tracer in the study of the physiology of the teeth. Science **106** (1947) 132. —⟨44⟩—.

[30] BASERGA, R. and K. NEMEROFF: The use of standard slides in semiquantitative radioautography with tritiated compounds. Stain Technol. **38** (1963) 111. —⟨156⟩—.

[31] BATISTINI, A., G. GIOVANNELLI and C. FAIENZA: On the nature of the thyroid hormone-binding protein. (Agar gel electrophoresis, immuno-electrophoresis, autoradiography). Lattante **33** (1962) 486. —⟨31⟩—.

[32] BECKER, S. and J. B. FRANCESCHINI: Track recognition system for scanning nuclear emulsions. IRE National Convention Record **9** (1957) 46. —⟨143⟩—.

[33] BÉLANGER, L. F.: A method for routine detection of radiophosphates and other radioactive compounds in tissues. The inverted autograph. Anat. Rec. **107** (1950) 149. —⟨79⟩—.

[34] BÉLANGER, L. F.: Improvements to the melted emulsion technique of autoradiography. Nature **170** (1952) 625. —⟨75⟩—.

[35] BÉLANGER, L. F.: Autoradiographic visualization of in vitro exchange in teeth, bones, and other tissues under various conditions. J. dent. Res. **32** (1953) 168 and Rev. Canad. Biol. **13** (1954) 52. —⟨44⟩—.

[36] BÉLANGER, L. F.: Autoradiographic detection of radiosulfate incorporation by the growing enamel of rats and hamsters. J. dent. Res. **34** (1955) 20. —⟨39⟩—.

[37] Bélanger, L. F.: The mineralization of rat enamel in the light of Ca^{45} autoradiography and microincineration. J. dent. Res. **36** (1957) 595. —⟨39⟩—.

[38] Bélanger, L. F.: Quantitative appreciation of comparative autoradiography of the synthesis and maintenance of some organic constituents of the epiphyseal plate of growing rats, in relation with magnesium deficiency. J. Histochem. Cytochem. **6** (1959) 146. —⟨161⟩—.

[39] Bélanger, L. F.: Alpharadiography: a simple method for determination of mass concentration in cells and tissues. J. biophys. biochem. Cytol. **6** (1959) 197. —⟨154⟩—.

[40] Bélanger, L. F. and C. P. Leblond: A method for locating radioactive elements in tissues by covering histological sections with a photographic emulsion. Endocrinology **39** (1946) 8. —⟨33, 75⟩—.

[41] Bélanger, L. F. and C. P. Leblond: Mineralization of the growing tooth as shown by radiophosphorus autographs. Proc. Soc. exp. Biol. (N. Y.) **73** (1950) 390. —⟨39⟩—.

[42] Bennington, J. L.: Radioautographic analysis of soluble antigen-antibody complexes separable by paper electrophoresis. Proc. Soc. exp. Biol. (N. Y.) **104** (1960) 148. —⟨32⟩—.

[43] Berlin, M., L.-G. Jerksell and G. Nordberg: Accelerated uptake of mercury by brain caused by 2.3 dimercaptopropanol (BAL) after injection into the mouse of a methyl-mercuric compound. Acta pharmacol. (Copenhagen) **23** (1965) 312. —⟨48⟩—.

[44] Berlin, M. and S. Ullberg: Accumulation and retention of mercury in the mouse. An autoradiographic study after a single intravenous injection of mercuric chloride. Arch. environm. Hlth. **6** (1963) 589. —⟨48⟩—.

[45] Berlin, M. and S. Ullberg: Accumulation and retention of mercury in the mouse. An autoradiographic comparison of phenyl mercuric acetate with inorganic mercury. Arch. environm. Hlth. **6** (1963) 602. —⟨48, 152⟩—.

[46] Berlin, M. and S. Ullberg: Accumulation and retention of mercury in the mouse. Autoradiographic comparison of methyl mercuric dicyanide diamide with inorganic mercury. Arch. environm. Hlth. **6** (1963) 610. —⟨48⟩—.

[47] Berlin, M. and S. Ullberg: Increased uptake of mercury in mouse brain caused by 2.3 dimercaptopropanol. Nature **197** (1964) 84. —⟨48, 49⟩—.

[48] Berriman, R. W., R. H. Herz and G. W. W. Stevens: A new photographic material — a high resolution emulsion for autoradiography. Brit. J. Radiol. **23** (1950) 472 and 578. —⟨61⟩—.

[49] Bhatnagar, A. S. and P. G. Ghosh: Using autoradiography for quantitative study of U in ore. Nucleonics **12/4** (1954) 58. —⟨158⟩—.

[50] Bierlein, T. K. and B. Mastel: Fission fragment damage in nonfissionable thin films. J. appl. Physics **31** (1960) 2315. —⟨122⟩—.

[51] Bierlein, T. K. and B. Mastel: Novel metallographic utilization of replicas and microautoradiography. Nucl. Sci. Abstr. **19** (1965) Abstr. No. 46951. —⟨22⟩—.

[52] Blanck, H., P. L. McCarthy and E. D. De Lamater: Novacuum freezing-dehydrating technic for histology, autoradiography, and microbial cytology. Stain Technol. **26** (1951) 193. —⟨78⟩—.

[53] Bleecken, S.: Quantitative Autoradiographie von tritiummarkierten Bakterien und Hefezellen. Atompraxis **10** (1964) 376. —⟨152⟩—.

[54] Bleecken, S.: The determination of autoradiographic resolution with ^{32}P-toned test images. Atompraxis **13** (1967) 190. —⟨72⟩—.

[55] BLEECKEN, S.: Die Methode der radioaktiven Tonung (insbesondere für ^{32}P) und ihre Anwendung in der Mikroautoradiographie für vergleichende Untersuchungen des Auflösungsvermögens. Atompraxis **14** (1968). —⟨72⟩—.

[56] BLEECKEN, S.: Die Abbildungseigenschaften autoradiographischer Systeme. I. Grundlagen zur Berechnung der autoradiographischen Übertragung. Z. Naturforsch. **23b** (1968) 1339. —⟨152⟩—.

[57] BLEECKEN, S.: Die Abbildungseigenschaften autoradiographischer Systeme. II. Lineare und nichtlineare autoradiographische Übertragung. Z. Naturforsch. **23b** (1968) 1350. —⟨152⟩—.

[58] BLEECKEN, S.: Die Abbildungseigenschaften autoradiographischer Systeme. III. Autoradiographisches Auflösungsvermögen. Z. Naturforsch. **23b** (1968) 1478. —⟨152⟩—.

[59] BODE, H. and J. EULER: Stromverteilung auf der Fläche von Akkuplatten. Naturwissenschaften **50** (1963) 610. —⟨20, 21⟩—.

[60] BOSQUE, P. G. and G. WERNER: Eine Methode zur radioautographischen Darstellung niedermolekularer und wasserlöslicher Stoffe in Organen. 2. Int. Kongr. Histochem. Cytochem., Frankfurt/M. 1964, p. 188. Springer-Verlag, Berlin-Göttingen-Heidelberg. —⟨79, 81⟩—.

[61] BOSTRÖM, R. C.: A projection microphotometer for quantitative microscopy. IRE Trans. Medical Electronics. PGME-7 (1956) 20. —⟨144⟩—.

[62] BOSTRÖM, H., E. ODEBLAD and U. FRIBERG: A quantitative autoradiographic study of the incorporation of S-35 in tracheal cartilage. Arch. Biochem. Biophysics **38** (1952) 283. —⟨161⟩—.

[63] BOSTRÖM, H., E. ODEBLAD and U. FRIBERG: A qualitative and quantitative autoradiographic study of the uptake of sulfur-35 labelled sodium sulfate in the skin of the adult rat. Acta path. microbiol. scand. **32** (1953) 516. —⟨161⟩—.

[64] BOVE, J. M.: Thin-layer chromatography and radioautography of adenosinephosphates in the presence of orthophosphate. Application to photosynthetic phosphorylation. Bull. Soc. Chim. biol. (Paris) **45** (1963) 421. —⟨29⟩—.

[65] BOYD, G. A. and H. LEVI: C-14 β-track autoradiography. Science **111** (1950) 58. —⟨142⟩—.

[66] BRÜCK, H. J.: Ein Beitrag zur Mikrophotographie ungefärbter Autoradiographie-Präparate. LEITZ-Mitt. Wiss. u. Techn. **IV/3** (1967) 83. —⟨74⟩—.

[67] BUBEL, H. C. and P. F. BONVENTRE: Apparatus for preparation of whole animal sections for autoradiography. J. Lab. Clin. Med. **61** (1963) 324. —⟨40, 44⟩—.

[68] BUCKALOV, G. W. and D. V. COHN: Color Autoradiography. Science **123** (1956) 333. —⟨30⟩—.

[69] BUDD, G. C.: Semi-quantitative electron autoradiography. In: 2. Internat. Kongr. Histochem. Cytochem., Frankfurt/M. 1964, p. 98. Springer-Verlag, Berlin-Göttingen-Heidelberg. —⟨157⟩—.

[70] BUDD, G. C. and S. R. PELC: The membrane method of electron microscope autoradiography. Stain Technol. **39** (1964) 295. —⟨103, 104⟩—.

[71] BUDD, G. C. and M. M. SALPETER: The distribution of labelled norepinephrine within sympathetic nerve terminals studied with electron microscope radioautography. J. Cell Biol. **41** (1969) 21. —⟨138⟩—.

[72] CAMPBELL, D.: Track autographs with iron-59 and sulphur-35 with quantitative evaluation. Nature **167** (1951) 274. —⟨142, 143⟩—.

[73] CAMPBELL, D. and B. H. PERSSON: Use of track autoradiography in studies on the sulfur metabolism of connective tissue. Experientia **7** (1951) 304. —⟨143, 161⟩—.

[74] Canny, M. J.: High resolution autoradiography of water-soluble substances. Nature **175** (1955) 857. —⟨69⟩—.

[75] Caro, L. G.: Proposed use of magnetic fields in electron microscopic radioautography. Nature **191** (1961) 1188. —⟨120⟩—.

[76] Caro, L. G.: Electron microscopic radioautography of thin sections: the Golgi zone as a site of protein concentration on pancreatic acinar cells. J. biophys. biochem. Cytol. **10** (1961) 37. —⟨109,128⟩—.

[77] Caro, L. G.: High-resolution autoradiography. II. The problem of resolution. J. Cell Biol. **15** (1962) 189. —⟨92⟩—.

[78] Caro, L. G.: High-resolution autoradiography. In: Methods in Cell Physiology. Vol. I, p. 327—363. Academic Press Inc., New York 1964. —⟨125, 126⟩—.

[79] Caro, L. G.: Progress in high-resolution autoradiography. Progr. Biophys. Mol. Biol. **16** (1966) 171. —⟨91⟩—.

[80] Caro, L. G. and G. E. Palade: Protein synthesis, storage, and discharge in the pancreatic exocrine cell. An autoradiographic study. J. Cell Biol. **20** (1964) 473. —⟨135, 137⟩—.

[81] Caro, L. G. and M. Schnoes: Tritium and phosphorus-32 in high resolution autoradiography. Science **149** (1965) 60. —⟨132⟩—.

[82] Caro, L. G and R. T. van Tubergen: High-resolution autoradiography. I. Methods. J. Cell Biol. **15** (1962) 173. —⟨100, 104, 106, 110, 116, 126, 127⟩—.

[83] Chamberlain, J., A. Hughes, A. W. Rogers and G. H. Thomas: An evaluation of the available techniques for the autoradiography of tritium on chromatograms. Nature **201** (1964) 774. —⟨24, 25, 26⟩—.

[84] Comings, D. E.: The duration of replication of the inactive X-chromosome in human based on the persistence of the heterochromatic sex chromatin body during DNA synthesis. Cytogenetics (Basel) **6** (1967) 20. —⟨68⟩—.

[85] Cormack, D. V.: Beta ray sensitivity of autoradiographic stripping film. Brit. J. Radiol. **28** (1955) 450. —⟨67, 70⟩—.

[86] Couceiro, A.: Deposicao do radiofosforo em tecidos osseo e dentario demonstrada pela tecnica autografica. Mem. Inst. Osw. Cruz, Rio de Janeiro **41** (1944) 541. —⟨44⟩—.

[87] La Cour, L. F. and J. W. C. Crawley: The site of rapidly labelled ribonucleic acid in nucleoli. Chromosoma (Berl.) **16** (1965) 124. —⟨135⟩—.

[88] Cupp, C. B. and P. Flubacher: Autoradiographic technique for the study of tritium in metals and its application to diffusion in zirconium at 149-deg. to 240-dge. C. J. nuclear Mater. (Amsterdam) **6** (1962) 213. —⟨16, 17, 18⟩—.

[89] Dalgaard, J. B.: Tracer phosphatase determination in tissue section. Nature **162** (1948) 811. —⟨160⟩—.

[90] Datta, N. P. and S. C. Srivastava: A method for radioautographic study of movement of phosphorus in soil columns. Nucl. Sci. Abstr. **13** (1959) Abstr. No. 6261. —⟨57⟩—.

[91] Davis, R. B. and D. Kay: Demonstration of 5-hydroxytryptamine in blood platelets by electron microscope autoradiography. Nature **207** (1965) 650. —⟨138⟩—.

[92] Debeauvais, M. and P. Cüer: Enregistrement des traces individuelles de particules α de faible énergie dans des films de nitrate de cellulose. C. R. Acad. Sci. (Paris) **258** (1964) 1777. —⟨122⟩—.

[93] v. DEIMLING, O., K. WITSCH and R. ROSSNER: Methoden zur nachträglichen PAS-und Feulgen-Färbung bei entwickelten autoradiographischen Paraffinschnitten. Histochemie **14** (1968) 242. —⟨77⟩—.

[94] DE MAN, J. C. H. and N. J. A. NOORDUYN: Light and electron microscopic radioautography of hepatic cell nucleoli in mice treated with actinomycin D. J. Cell Biol. **33** (1967) 489. —⟨133⟩—.

[95] DENDY, P. P.: A method for the automatic estimation of grain densities in microautoradiography. Phys. in Med. Biol. **5** (1960) 131. —⟨145⟩—.

[96] DENNIS, E. S. and R. G. WAKE: Autoradiography of the *Bacillus subtilis* chromosome. J. molec. Biol. **15** (1966) 435. —⟨65, 66⟩—.

[97] DESCARRIES, L. and B. DROZ: Electron microscope radioautographic detection of norepinephrine-H^3 in the central nervous system of the rat. In: Electron Microscopy 1968, Vol. II, p. 527 (Rome 1968). — ⟨138⟩—.

[98] DESCARRIES, L. and B. DROZ: Incorporation de noradrénaline-^3H(NA-^3H) dans le système nerveux central du rat adulte. Etude radio-autographique en microscopie électronique. C. R. Acad. Sci. (Paris) Serie D **266** (1968) 2480. —⟨138⟩—.

[99] DESSAUER, H. C., W. FOX and Q. L. HARTWIG: Comparative study of transferrins of amphibia and reptilia using starch-gel electrophoresis and autoradiography. Comp. Biochem. Physiol. **5** (1962) 17. — ⟨31, 32⟩ —.

[100] DEUCHAR, E. M.: Staining sections before autoradiographic exposure. Excessive background graining caused by celestin blue. Stain Technol. **37** (1962) 324. — ⟨68⟩ —.

[101] DOCKUM, N. L. and J. W. HEALY: Spot diameter method of quantitative autoradiography of ruthenium-106 particles in lung tissues. Stain Technol. **32** (1957) 209. — ⟨142, 143⟩ —.

[102] DÖRMER, P.: Auflichtphotometrische Untersuchungen zur Größe der Koinzidenz in der Autoradiographie mit Tritium. Histochemie **8** (1967) 1. — ⟨150⟩ —.

[103] DÖRMER, P.: Erfahrungen mit der photometrischen Silberkornzählung in der Autoradiographie. LEITZ-Mitt. Wiss. u. Techn. **IV/3** (1967) 74. — ⟨145⟩ —.

[104] DÖRMER, P., W. BRINKMANN, A. STIEBER and W. STICH: Automatische Silberkornzählung in der Einzelzell-Autoradiographie. Eine neue photometrische Methode für die quantitative Autoradiographie. Klin. Wschr. **44** (1966) 477. — ⟨145, 146⟩ —.

[105] DOHLMAN, G. F. and J. FARKASHIDY: Evaluation of different methods of autoradiography in electron microscopy. 5th Intern. Congr. Electron Microscr. Philadelphia, Vol. II (1962) 1—11. — ⟨116⟩ — .

[106] DOHLMAN, G. F., A. B. MAUNSBACH, L. HAMMARSTRÖM and L. E. APPELGREN: Electron microscopic autoradiography. A method for producing monolayers of silver halide crystals using centrifuge sedimentation. J. Ultrastruct. Res. **10** (1964) 293. — ⟨116⟩ —.

[107] DOMINGUES, F. J., A. SARKO and R. R. BALDWIN: A simplified method for quantitation of autoradiography. Int. J. appl. Radiat. **1** (1956) 94. — ⟨152⟩ —.

[108] DONIACH, J. and S. R. PELC: Autoradiograph technique. Brit. J. Radiol. **23** (1950) 184. — ⟨92⟩ —.

[109] DROZ, M. B.: Biologie cellulaire. Sites de synthèse et migration des protéines dans les cellules hépatiques du Rat: étude radioautographique en microscopie électronique. C. R. Acad. Sci. (Paris) Série D **262** (1966) 1654. — ⟨135, 158⟩ —.

[110] DROZ, M. B.: Biologie Cellulaire. Elaboration de glycoprotéines dans l'appareil de Golgi des cellules hépatiques chez le Rat; étude radioautographique en

microscopie électronique après injection de galactose-^{3}H. C. R. Acad. Sci. (Paris) Série D **262** (1966) 1766. — ⟨135, 158⟩ —.

[111] Droz, B. and M. Bergeron: Radioautographic detection of proteins newly synthesized from leucine-H-3 in the mitochondria of the liver and kidney of the rat. C. R. Acad. Sci. (Paris) **261** (1965) 2757 (French). — ⟨135⟩ —.

[112] Droz, B. and M. Bergeron: Quantitative electron microscopic radioautography: conditions and application to the kinetics of mitochondrial proteins. Electron Microscopy and Cytochemistry, Symposium Leiden 1966. — ⟨158⟩ —.

[113] Droz, B., H. L. Koenig and R. W. Young: Radioautographie en microscopie électronique et renouvellement des protéines axonales dans les terminaisons motrices et sénsitives. In: Electron Microscopy, Vol. II/1968, p. 523 (Rome 1968). — ⟨135⟩ —.

[114] Dudley, R. A. and M. B. Dobyns: Use of autoradiographs in quantitative determination of radiation dosages from Ca^{45} in bone. Science **109** (1948) 327. — ⟨161⟩ —.

[115] Dudley, R. A. and S. R. Pelc: Automatic grain counter for assessing quantitatively high-resolution autoradiographs. Nature **172** (1953) 992. — ⟨147⟩ —.

[116] Duhm, B., W. Maul, H. Medenwald, K. Patzschke and L. A. Wegner: Tierexperimentelle Untersuchungen mit radioaktiv markiertem α-Methyldopa. Naunyn-Schmiedeberg's Arch. exp. Path. Pharmak. **246** (1963) 10. — ⟨46, 47⟩ —

[117] Duhm, B., W. Maul, H. Medenwald, K. Patzschke and L. A. Wegner: Autoradiographische Studien über die Verteilung von α-Methyldopa in der Ratte und im Katzenhirn. Atompraxis **10** (1964) 46. — ⟨46⟩ —.

[118] Dumcombe, W. G.: A nomogram for calculating autoradiograph exposures. Int. J. appl. Radiat. **10** (1961) 212. — ⟨156, 157⟩ —.

[119] Eckert, H. and A. Hopf: Autoradiographic studies on the distribution of psychoactive drugs in the rat brain. Int. Pharmocopsychiat. **2** (1969) 12. — ⟨151⟩ —.

[120] Edström, A.: Inhibition of protein synthesis in Mauthner nerve fibre components by Actinomycin-D. J. Neurochem. **14** (1967) 239. — ⟨133⟩ —.

[121] Elfvin, L. E., L. E. Applegren and S. Ullberg: High-resolution autoradiography of the adrenal medulla after injection of tritiated dihydroxyphenylalanine (Dopa). J. Ultrastruct. Res. **14** (1966) 277. — ⟨138⟩ —.

[122] Endicott, K. M. and H. Yagoda: Microscopic historadiographic technic for locating and quantitating radioactive elements in tissues. Proc. Soc. exp. Biol. (N. Y.) **64** (1947).170. — ⟨45⟩ —.

[123] Erbacher, D. and E. Wannemacher: Zur Frage von Stoffwechselvorgängen in den Zahnhartgeweben. Dtsch. Zahn-, Mund- und Kieferheilk. **8** (1941) 201. — ⟨44⟩ —.

[124] Erickson, W. H. and D. Hardie: The autoradiographic location of precipitated hydride in a Zr-2% Nb alloy. J. Inst. Metals **92** (1964) 191. — ⟨16⟩ —.

[125] Erismann, K. H.: Hilfsmittel zum Arbeiten mit radioaktiven Substanzen in der Dünnschichtchromatographie. J. Chromatog. **20** (1965) 600. — ⟨26⟩ —.

[126] Ertraud, E. and P. Zaleski: Neutron density measurements by autoradiography of detector foils. J. Phys. Radium (Paris) **14** (1953) 191. — ⟨158⟩ —.

[127] Euler, J.: Verwendung von Radioisotopen in der Batterie-Forschung. Chemie-Ing.-Techn. **38** (1966) 631. — ⟨19⟩ —.

[128] Evans, T. C.: Radioautographs in which the tissue is mounted directly on the photographic plate. Proc. Soc. Exp. Biol. (N. Y.) **64** (1947) 313. — ⟨33, 45⟩ —.

[129] Faraggi, H.: Some examples of the use of autoradiography in metallurgy. Nucl. Sci. Abstr. **14** (1960) Abstr. No. 4713. — ⟨10⟩ —.

[130] Feinendegen, L. E.: Zusammenfassende Übersichten zu den Versuchen der autoradiographischen Darstellung leichtlöslicher Substanzen. Acta histochem. Jena, Suppl. VIII (1968) 107. — ⟨78⟩ —.

[131] Fewer, D., J. Threadgold and H. Sheldon: Studies on cartilage. V. Electron microscopic observations on the autoradiographic localization of S-35 in cells and matrix. J. Ultrastruct. Res. **11** (1964) 166. — ⟨111, 135⟩ —.

[132] Field, E. O., K. B. Dawson and J. E. Gibbs: Autoradiographic differentiation of tritium and another β-emitter by a combined color-coupling and double stripping-film technique. Stain Technol. **40** (1965) 295. — ⟨64⟩ —.

[133] Field, E. O., K. B. Dawson and G. W. W. Stevens: Differential autoradiography of tritium and another β-emitter by a double stripping-film technique. Nature **195** (1962) 510. — ⟨64⟩ —.

[134] Firket, H. and P. Granboulan: Electron microscope autoradiographs of tritiated uridine incorporation. J. roy. micr. Soc. **81** (1963) 227. — ⟨135⟩ —.

[135] Fischer, H. A. and G. Werner: Eine Methode zur quantitativen Auswertung von Autoradiogrammen auf der Grundlage der Durchlicht-Mikro-Photometrie. Histochemie **15** (1968) 84. — ⟨89, 150, 151, 152⟩ —.

[136] Fischer, H. A. and G. Werner: Untersuchungen zur Eignung photographischer Emulsionen für die elektronenmikroskopische Autoradiographie. Acta histochem. (Jena) Suppl. VIII (1968) 155. — ⟨99, 123, 125⟩ —.

[137] Fischer, H. A. and G. Werner: Apparative Anordnung zur histologischen und quantitativen Analyse von Autoradiogrammen. Z. analyt. Chem. **243** (1968) 183. — ⟨90, 152⟩ —.

[138] Fitzgerald, J. P., E. Simmel, J. Weinstein and C. Martin: Radioautography: Theory, technic, and applications. Lab. Invest. **2** (1953) 181. — ⟨79⟩ —.

[139] Flinn, M.: Calculation of exposure times for successive autoradiographs. Nature **202** (1964) 1036. — ⟨157⟩ —.

[140] Fodor, J.: Some uses of autoradiography in the metallurgical industry. Energia és Atomtechn. **12** (1959) 275 and Nucl. Sci. Abstr. **14** (1960) Abstr. No. 15030. — ⟨10⟩ —.

[141] Foster, L. M., A. S. jr. Gillespie, T. H. Jack and W. W. Hill: Hydrogen in aluminium-tritium autoradiography. Nucleonics **21/4** (1963) 53. — ⟨16⟩ —.

[142] Fray, G. and J. Frey: Highly sensitive radioautographic technique to be used for thin-layer chromatography. Bull. Soc. Chim. biol. **45** (1963) 1201. — ⟨28⟩ —.

[143] Fromme, H. G.: Ein Beitrag zur Methodik der elektronenmikroskopischen Autoradiographie. Z. Naturforsch. **19b** (1964) 852. — ⟨106⟩ —.

[144] Fromme, H. G., W. Stöber and F. J. Strecker: Elektronenmikroskopisch-autoradiographische Lokalisierung von subkutan injiziertem Poly-vinyl-pyridin-N-oxid in Tridymitstaub-Granulomen von Ratten. Hoppe-Seyler's Z. physiol. Chem. **346** (1966) 74. — ⟨138⟩ —.

[145] Fromme, H. G. and U. Zessack: Electron microscopic autoradiography in a magnetic field. Electron microscopy and Cytochemistry Symposium Leiden 1966. — ⟨120⟩ —.

[146] Fujita, H. and S. Fujita: Electron microscopic studies on neuroblast differentiation in the central nervous system of domestic fowl. Z. Zellforsch. **60** (1963) 463. — ⟨135⟩ —.

[147] Fujita, H. and S. Fujita: Electron microscopic studies on the differentiation of the ependymal cells and the glioblast in the spinal cord of domestic fowl. Z. Zellforsch. **64** (1964) 262. — ⟨135⟩ —.
[148] Gabler, F.: Microphotometry and its application. The Microscope & Crystal Front **15** (1966) 85. — ⟨145⟩ —.
[149] Gardiner, J. R.: A radioactive marking ink. Nature **197** (1963) 414. — ⟨23⟩ —.
[150] Garweg, G. and H. Kortmann: Die infundibulären Zonen der normalen und adrenalektomierten weißen Maus in der Kryostat- und Paraffinschnitt-Autoradiographie. Z. Zellforsch. **92** (1968) 94. — ⟨81⟩ —.
[151] v. Gaudecker, B.: Elektronenmikroskopische Autoradiographie mit H^3-Thymidin an der Thymusrinde der Maus. Z. Zellforsch. **72** (1966) 281. — ⟨135⟩ —.
[152] George II, L. A. and G. S. Vogt: Electron microscopy of autoradiographed radioactive particles. Nature **184** (1959) 1474. — ⟨104, 106⟩ —.
[153] Getsel, A. Kh.: A simplified method of using standards for quantitative autoradiography. Biofizika **6** (1961) 219 (Russian); English translation in: Biophysics **6** (1961) 240. — ⟨152⟩ —.
[154] Geuskens, M. and A. Ficq: Detection of DNA by a autoradiographic method after "staining" with radioactive Actinomycin D and high-resolution autoradiography. Acta Histochem. (Jena) Suppl. VIII, (1968) 135. — ⟨133⟩ —.
[155] Ghiara, G.: Attivita di sintesi proteica econstituzione di granuli di secrezione: ricerche istoautoradiografiche e di microscopia elettronica sul pancreas esocrino. Boll. Zool. **29** (1962) 73. — ⟨132⟩ —.
[156] Glawitsch, G.: Über die Anwendung radioaktiver Methoden auf metallkundliche Probleme (Autoradiographie). Z. Metallkunde **47** (1956) 199. — ⟨10, 11, 14⟩ —.
[157] Gleason, G. J., D. J. Taylor and D. L. Tabern: Absolute beta counting at defined geometry. Nucleonics **8/5** (1951) 12. — ⟨6⟩ —.
[158] Godman, G. C. and N. Lane: On the site of sulfation in the chondrocyte. J. Cell. Biol. **21** (1964) 353. — ⟨135⟩ —.
[159] Goldin, M. L., U. I. Krivonosov, G. N. Kovalev, F. E. Dolzhenkov and M. B. Tobolskii: Use of an autoradiographic method for the study of the boundary zone of bimetals. Zadvodsk. Lab. **31** (1965) 230. — ⟨10⟩ —.
[160] Gomberg, H. J., M. J. Simott, C. Upthegrove, R. A. Flinn, L. H. van Vlack, S. Yukawa, A. S. Keh, H. B. Probst, C. M. Hammond, R. Simonsen and G. C. Towe: High-resolution autoradiography for study of grain boundaries in metals. Final report. Nucl. Sci. Abstr. **8** (1954) Abstr. No. 4290. — ⟨10⟩ —.
[161] Gordon, B. E. and V. K. Lisichenko: An autoradiographic method of examining pencil and ink mark on documents. Int. J. appl. Radiat. **8** (1960) 138. — ⟨51, 52⟩ —.
[162] Granboulan, P.: Resolving power and sensitivity of a new emulsion in electron microscope autoradiography. J. roy. micr. Soc. (Ser. 3) **81** (1963) 165. — ⟨100⟩ —.
[163] Granboulan, P. and R. Audran: Application of Lippmann-type emulsion to autoradiography with an electron microscope. C. R. Acad. Sci. (Paris) **259** (1964) 3201. — ⟨100⟩ —.
[164] Granboulan, P., N. Granboulan and W. Bernhard: Application de l'autoradiographie à la Microscopie Electronique. J. de Microscopie **1** (1962) 75. — ⟨116, 134⟩ —.

[165] Granboulan, N. and P. Tournier: Horaire et localisation de la synthèse des acides nucléiques pendant la phase d'éclipse du virus SV 40. Ann. Inst. Pasteur (Paris) **109** (1965) 837. — ⟨134⟩ —.

[166] Grennen Tsuk, R., Th. Castro, L. Laufer and D. R. Schwarz: Determination of radiochemical purity by means of autoradiography. In: Proc. Conf. Methods of Preparing and Storing Marked Molecules, Brussels 1963, p. 497—509. — ⟨25⟩ —.

[167] Grosskreutz, J. C.: Autoradiography of fatigue fracture in aluminium. J. appl. Physics. **33** (1962) 2653. — ⟨15⟩ —.

[168] Grunberg, L.: The formation of hydrogen peroxide on fresh metal surfaces. Proc. phys. Soc. B 66 (1953) 153. — ⟨15⟩ —.

[169] Gude, W. D.: Controlled humidity of autoradiographic stripping film during storage. Stain Technol. **32** (1957) 197. — ⟨63⟩ —.

[170] Guidotti, G.: Quantitative autoradiography of isolated thyroid-gland colloid. Stain Technol. **31** (1956) 7. — ⟨161⟩ —.

[171] Guidotti, G. and R. L. Setti: Autoradiography of tracks from β-particle emitters in tissues. Stain Technol. **31** (1956) 57. — ⟨142⟩ —.

[172] Guilbert, J. M. and J. A. S. Adams: Alpha-particle autoradiography with liquid emulsion. Nucleonics **13/7** (1955) 43. — ⟨142⟩ —.

[173] Gullberg, J. E.: A new change-over optical system and a direct recording microscope for quantitative autoradiography. Exp. Cell Res. Suppl. **4** (1957) 222. — ⟨145⟩ —.

[174] Gullberg, J. E.: Grain counting instrumentation. Lab. Invest. 8 (1959) 94. — ⟨144⟩ —.

[175] Guroff, G.: The hydroxylation-induced migration of tritium: Practical Aspects. Atomlight **69** (1969) 1. — ⟨9⟩ —.

[176] Haase, G. and G. Jung: Herstellung von Einkornschichten aus photographischen Emulsionen. Naturwissenschaften **51** (1964) 404. — ⟨106, 107, 130⟩ —.

[177] Hamilton, J. G.: The metabolism of the fission products and the heaviest elements. Radiology **49** (1947) 325. — ⟨40⟩ —.

[178] Hamm, F. A. and J. J. Comer: Electron microscopy of photographic grains. Specimen preparation techniques and applications. J. appl. Physics **24** (1953) 1495. — ⟨91⟩ —.

[179] Hammarström, L.: Autoradiographic studies on C^{14}-labelled ascorbic acid and dehydroascorbic acid. Acta physiol. scand. **70** (1966) Suppl. 289. — ⟨46⟩ —.

[180] Hampton, J. C. and H. Quastler: Combined autoradiography and electron microscopy of thin sections of intestinal epithelial cells of the mouse labelled with thymidine. J. biophys. biochem. Cytol. **10** (1961) 140. — ⟨104, 106, 134⟩ —.

[181] Harbers, E.: Untersuchungen über Verteilung und Ausscheidung der in vivo entstehenden Folgeprodukte des Thorium X. Z. Naturforsch. **7b** (1952) 365. — ⟨143⟩ —.

[182] Harford, C. G. and A. Hamlin: Electron microscopic autoradiography in a magnetic field. Nature **189** (1961) 505. — ⟨120⟩ —.

[183] Harford, C. G. and A. Hamlin: A method of electron microscopic autoradiography with tritium-labelled cells in a magnetic field. Lab. Invest. **10** (1961) 627. — ⟨120⟩ —.

[184] Harris, J. E., J. F. Sloane and D. T. King: New techniques in autoradiography. Nature **166** (1950) 25. — ⟨69, 142⟩ —.

[185] HAY, E. D. and J. P. REVEL: The fine structure of the DNP component of the nucleus. An electron microscopic study utilizing autoradiography to localize DNA synthesis. J. Cell Biol. **16** (1963) 29. — ⟨111⟩ —.
[186] HELLAUER, H. and K. HAGEMÜLLER: Zur quantitativen Bestimmung der Jodeiweißbindung im Gewebe auf radiohistochemischer Basis. Strahlentherapie, Sonderband **38** (1958) 82. — ⟨31, 32, 128⟩ —.
[187] HERRMANN, W.: Untersuchungen an Bleibatterien mit der Isotopen-Indikatormethode. Elektrotechn. Z. **B16** (1964) 643. — ⟨19⟩ —.
[188] HERRMANN, W., G. HARTMANN, K.-H. BOTHE and G. HOFMANN: A micro-autoradiographic method for detection of the distribution of silicic acid of filler in rubber. Kernenergie **3** (1960) 663. — ⟨56⟩ —.
[189] HERRMANN, W., G. HARTMANN and R. BRUST: Das Auflösungsvermögen mikroautoradiographischer Aufnahmen in Abhängigkeit von der Energie der verwendeten β-Strahlung (Teil I). Atompraxis **7** (1961) 315. — ⟨72, 92⟩ —.
[190] HERRMANN, W., G. HARTMANN and R. BRUST: Das Auflösungsvermögen mikroautoradiographischer Aufnahmen und Untersuchungen über seine Abhängigkeit von der Energie der verwendeten β-Strahlung. (Teil II). Atompraxis **8** (1962) 8. — ⟨172⟩ —.
[191] HERRMANN, W. and G. PRÖBSTL: Versuche über die Antimonverteilung im Bleiakkumulator. Z. Elektrochem., Ber. Bunsenges. physik. Chem. **61** (1957) 1157. — ⟨19⟩ —.
[192] HERZ, R. H.: Photographic fundamentals of autoradiography. Nucleonics **9** (1951) 24. — ⟨71⟩ —.
[193] HERZ, R. H.: Micro-Autoradiographie. Röntgenblätter **9** (1956) 201. — ⟨72⟩ —.
[194] HERZ, R. H.: Methods to improve the performance of stripping emulsions. Lab. Invest. 8 (1959) 71. — ⟨71, 76, 124⟩ —.
[195] HILL, D. K.: Resolving power with tritium autoradiographs. Nature **194** (1962) 831. — ⟨152⟩ —.
[196] HILSCHER, B., W. HILSCHER and W. MAURER: Autoradiographische Bestimmung der Generationszeiten und Teilphasen der verschiedenen Spermatogonien-Generationen der Ratte. Naturwissenschaften **53** (1966) 415. — ⟨162⟩ —.
[197] HILSCHER, W. and W. MAURER: Autoradiographische Bestimmung der Dauer der DNS-Verdopplung und ihres zeitlichen Verlaufs bei Spermatogonien der Ratte durch Doppelmarkierung mit C-14- und H-3-Thymidin. Naturwissenschaften **49** (1962) 352. — ⟨162⟩ —.
[198] HOECKER, F. E. and P. G. ROOFE: Structural differences in bone matrix associated with metabolized radium. Radiology **52** (1949) 856. — ⟨89⟩ —.
[199] HOLGATE, W.: The incorporation and retention of Sr^{90} in the teeth. Brit. dent. J. **107** (1959) 131. — ⟨39⟩ —.
[200] HOLMSEN, H.: Incorporation in vitro of P^{32} into blood platelet acid-soluble organophosphates and their chromatographic identification. Scand. J. clin. Lab. Invest. **17** (1965) 230. — ⟨25⟩ —.
[201] HOLT, S. J. and R. M. HICKS: Specific staining methods for enzyme localization at the subcellular level. Brit. med. Bull. **18** (1962) 214. — ⟨133⟩ —.
[202] HOLT, M. W. and SH. WARREN: A radioautographic method for detailed localization of radioactive isotopes in tissues without isotope loss. Proc. Soc. Exp. Biol. (N. Y.) **73** (1950) 545. — ⟨23, 89⟩ —.
[203] HOREŠOVSKY, O., J. DUPAL and I. M. HAIS: A frame for photographic processing of the autoradiograms of paper chromatograms or electrophorograms. J. Chromatogr. **9** (1962) 260. — ⟨26⟩ —.

[204] Howard, A. and S. R. Pelc: Synthesis of deoxyribosenucleic acid and nuclear incorporation of S-35 as shown by autoradiography. Ciba Found. Conf. Isotope in Biochemistry **1951**, p. 138—151. — ⟨162⟩ —.

[205] Howard, A. and S. R. Pelc: Synthesis of nucleoprotein in bean root cells. Nature **167** (1951) 599. — ⟨162⟩ —.

[206] Howard, A. and S. R. Pelc: Nuclear Incorporation of P^{32} as demonstrated by Autoradiographs. Exp. Cell Res. **2** (1951) 178. — ⟨162⟩ —.

[207] Howard, A. and S. R. Pelc: Synthesis of deoxyribonucleic acid in normal and irradiated cells and its relation to chromosome breakage. Heredity **6** (1953) Suppl., 261. — ⟨162⟩ —.

[208] Hsieh, J. J. C., F. P. Hungate and S. A. Wilson: Autoradiography: Technique for drastic reduction of exposure time to alpha particles. Science **150** (1965) 1821. — ⟨43⟩ —.

[209] Huettig, G. F. and G. Glawitsch: Autoradiographic methods in powder metallurgy. Powder Met. Bull. **7** (1956) 108. — ⟨10⟩ —.

[210] Hug, O. and O. Balk: Patent: 3-H, Empfindlichkeitserhöhung im elektrischen Feld. Atompraxis **8** (1962) 281. — ⟨121⟩ —.

[211] Hughes, W. L., V. P. Bond, G. Brecher, E. P. Cronkite, R. B. Painter, H. Quastler and F. G. Sherman: Cellular proliferation in the mouse as revealed by autoradiography with tritiated thymidine. Proc. nat. Acad. Sci. (Wash.) **44** (1958) 476. — ⟨71⟩ —.

[212] Isbell, H. S., H. L. Frush and R. A. Peterson: J. Res. Nat. Bur. Standards A **63** (1959) 171. — ⟨26⟩ —.

[213] Jackson, R.: Autoradiography of electrophoretic starch gels containing Fe^{59}. J. biol. photogr. Ass. **27** (1959) 49. — ⟨31, 32⟩ —.

[214] Jodrey, L. H. and K. M. Wilbur: Autoradiograms of irregular surfaces. Proc. Soc. exp. Biol. **77** (1951) 80. — ⟨58⟩ —.

[215] Joftes, D. L.: Liquid emulsion autoradiography with tritium. Lab. Invest. **8** (1959) 131. — ⟨76⟩ —.

[216] Joftes, D. L.: Radioautography, principles, and procedures. J. Nucl. Med. **4** (1963) 143. — ⟨76⟩ —.

[217] Joftes, D. L. and Sh. Warren: Simplified liquid emulsion radioautography. J. biol. photogr. Ass. **23** (1955) 145. — ⟨76⟩ —.

[218] Johnson, P., E. J. Weber, H. E. Carter and M. S. Krober: Detection of phospholipids on paper chromatograms by neutron activation. J. Lipid. Res. **6** (1965) 425. — ⟨25⟩ —.

[219] Johnston, W. B.: Autoradiography of soil sections and its applications. Soil Science **78** (1954) 247. — ⟨57⟩. —.

[220] Jowsey, J.: Densitometry of photographic images. J. appl. Physiol. **21** (1966) 309. — ⟨144⟩ —.

[221] Jowsey, J., B. A. Lafferty and J. Rabinowitz: Analysis of distribution of Ca^{45} in dog bone by a quantitative autoradiographic method. J. Bone Jt. Surg. A. **47** (1965) 359. — ⟨161⟩ —.

[222] Kalberer, F.: A new method of macro-autoradiography. Atomlight **51** (1966) 1 and Adv. Trac. Meth. **3** (1966) 139. — ⟨42, 45⟩ —.

[223] Kaminski, E. J.: Histologic processing in autoradiography: Loss of radioactivity. Stain Technol. **30** (1955) 139. — ⟨68⟩ —.

[224] Karasaki, S.: Electron microscopic examination of the sites of nuclear RNA synthesis during amphibian embryogenesis. J. Cell Biol. **26** (1965) 937. — ⟨135⟩ —.

[225] Kastenbaum, M. A. and M. G. Hanna jr.: Statistical analysis of autoradiographic and histologic data. Arch. Path. (Chicago) **79** (1965) 462. — ⟨155⟩ —.

[226] Kayes, J., A. B. Maunsbach and S. Ullberg: Electron microscopic autoradiography of radioiodine in the thyroid using the extranuclear electrons of I-125. J. Ultrastruct. Res. **7** (1962) 339. — ⟨128, 137⟩ —.

[227] Kennedy, G. D. C. and J. S. Kennedy: An autoradiographic study of the dental lesions of lathyrism in the rat. Arch. oral. Biol. **8** (1963) 207. — ⟨39⟩ —.

[228] Kinersly, T.: Beta-track autoradiographic study of teeth with Ca^{45}. Yale J. Biol. Med. **27** (1954) 114. — ⟨39⟩ —.

[229] King, D. T., J. E. Harris and S. Tkackzyk: Liquid emulsion methods in electron track autoradiography. Nature **167** (1951) 273. — ⟨142⟩ —.

[230] Kirshenbaum, A. D., C. W. Hoffman and A. V. Grosse: Autoradiographic technique with carbon-14 in rubber. Analytic. Chem. **23** (1951) 1440. — ⟨54, 55, 56⟩ —.

[231] Kisieleski, W. E., R. Baserga and J. Vaupotic: The efficiency of autoradiographic stripping-film applied to tissue sections containing tritiated thymidine. Radiat. Res. **15** (1962) 341 and Adv. Trac. Meth. **1** (1963) 302. — ⟨71⟩ —.

[232] Klein, E.: Electronmicroscopic investigations of photographic layers. Photogr. Sci. Engng. **1** (1957) 52. — ⟨97⟩ —.

[233] Koburg, E. and W. Maurer: Autoradiographische Untersuchungen mit H^3-Thymidin über die Dauer der Desoxyribonukleinsäure-Synthese und ihrem zeitlichen Verlauf bei den Darmepithelien und anderen Zelltypen der Maus. Biochim. biophys. Acta (Amst.) **61** (1962) 229. — ⟨162⟩ —.

[234] KODAK-firm prospectus: Scientific and technical data P-64, 2nd Ed. 1966. KODAK-materials for nuclear physics and autoradiography. — ⟨67⟩ —.

[235] Koehler, J. K., K. Mühlethaler and A. Frey-Wyssling: Electron microscopic autoradiography. An improved technique for producing thin films and its application to H-3-thymidine-labeled maize nuclei. J. Cell Biol. **16** (1963) 73. — ⟨114, 115, 135⟩ —.

[236] Kohlhörster, J.: Beiträge zur Bestimmung kleinster Alpha-Aktivitäten mit Hilfe der photographischen Bahnspurdarstellung. Strahlentherapie **94** (1954) 602. — ⟨143⟩ —.

[237] Kominek, J. and M. Radwin: Method of thickness determination of metallographic specimens for autoradiography. Nukleonika **10** (1965) 62. — ⟨10⟩ —.

[238] Kopriwa, B. M.: Demonstration of coating technique for electron microscopic radioautography. Anat. Rec. **151** (1965) 490 (Abstract). — ⟨111⟩ —.

[239] Kopriwa, B. M.: A semiautomatic instrument for the radioautographic coating technique. J. Histochem. Cytochem. **14** (1966) 923. — ⟨104, 111, 112⟩ —.

[240] Kopriwa, B. M. and C. P. Leblond: Improvements in the coating technique of radioautography. J. Histochem. Cytochem. **10** (1962) 269. — ⟨76, 78⟩ —.

[241] Kumamoto, Y. and C. P. Leblond: Radioautographic study of mineralization of growing teeth with labeled calcium. J. dent. Res. **35** (1956) 147. — ⟨39⟩ —.

[242] Kutzim, H.: Quantitative autoradiographische Untersuchungen an Ganztierschnitten zum Mineralstoffwechsel (Jod, Phosphor, Schwefel und Kupfer). Verh. dtsch. Ges. Path. **46** (1962) 243. — ⟨149⟩ —.

[243] Kutzim, H.: The quantitative determination of the distribution of S-35-sulfate in mice using autoradiography. Nucl. Med. **3** (1962) 39. — ⟨161⟩ —.

[244] KUTZIM, H.: Quantitative Stoffwechseluntersuchungen mit Hilfe der Autoradiographie. Elektromedizin **7** (1962) 220. — ⟨161⟩ —.

[245] KUTZIM, H.: Quantitative Untersuchungen über die Verteilung von J^{131} und Cu^{64} mit Hilfe von Ganztierschnitten. Acta histochem. (Jena) Suppl. **3** (1963) 233. — ⟨149⟩ —.

[246] LAJTHA, L. G. and R. OLLIVER: The application of autoradiography in the study of nucleic acid metabolism. Lab. Invest. **8** (1959) 214. — ⟨71⟩ —.

[247] LAL, H.: Distribution of urease activity in mice studied by whole-animal autoradiography. Int. J. appl. Radiat. **15** (1964) 543. — ⟨49⟩ —.

[248] LAMBIOTTE, M.: Physicochimie biologique. — Un nouveau procédé de séperation et de détection des substances tritiées: l'électrophorèse autoradiographique en couche mince de gélatine photographique. C. R. Acad. Sci. (Paris) **260** (1965) 1799. — ⟨30⟩ —.

[249] LAMBIOTTE, M.: Autoradiographic electrophoresis of tritium labeled compounds in a thin layer of buffered photographic gelatine. Nature **207** (1965) 516. — ⟨30⟩ —.

[250] LAMBIOTTE, M.: Thin layer autoradiographic electrophoresis of tritium-labelled compounds in buffered photographic gelatine. Adv. Trac. Meth. **3** (1966) 157. — ⟨30⟩ —.

[251] LAMERTON, L. F. and E. B. HARRISS: Some autoradiographic studies of non-uniform distribution of radioactive phosphorus in tissues. Brit. Med. J. Vol. II (1951) 932. — ⟨71⟩ —.

[252] LANG, W. and W. MAURER: Zur Verwendbarkeit von Feulgen-gefärbten Schnitten für quantitative Autoradiographie mit markiertem Thymidin. Exp. Cell Res. **39** (1965) 1. — ⟨68⟩ —.

[253] LAUDE, P. P., R. G. JANES and J. D. BOYD: A simplified machine for making ground sections of teeth or bone. Anat. Rec. **104** (1949) 11. — ⟨38⟩ —.

[254] LEBLOND, C. P. and K. B. WARREN: The use of radioautography in investigating protein synthesis. Symp. Int. Soc. Cell Biol. 1965/IV, Academic Press Inc. New York and London. — ⟨163⟩ —.

[255] LEDER, O.: Autoradiographic studies on the distribution of P^{32}-labelled orthophosphates in whole animal body sections. Pflüger's Arch. ges. Physiol. **276** (1962) 250. — ⟨47⟩ —.

[256] LELENTAL, E. and A. SZUCHNIK: Detection of fingerprints by autoradiography. (Initial report). Int. J. appl. Radiat. **15** (1964) 373. — ⟨54⟩ —.

[257] LENNARTZ, K. J. and W. MAURER: Autoradiographische Bestimmung der Dauer der DNS-Verdoppelung und der Generationszeit beim Ehrlich-Ascitestumor der Maus durch Doppelmarkierung mit C^{14}- und H^3-Thymidin. Z. Zellforsch. **63** (1964) 478. — ⟨162⟩ —.

[258] LENNARTZ, K. J., W. MAURER and N. SCHÜMMELFEDER: Die DNS-Verdopplungszeit und Generationsdauer beim Ehrlich-Ascitestumor der Maus. Verh. dtsch. Ges. Path. **1964**, 280—288. — ⟨162⟩ —.

[259] LESCH, R., W. SCHIESSLE and W. OEHLERT: Autoradiographische Untersuchungen zur DNS-Synthese an menschlichem Exzisionsmaterial aus dem Bronchialbaum. Beitr. path. Anat. **129** (1964) 296. — ⟨161⟩ —.

[260] LETTRÉ, H. and N. PAWELETZ: Probleme der elektronenmikroskopischen Autoradiographie. Naturwissenschaften **53** (1966) 268. — ⟨128, 130⟩ —.

[261] LEVI, H.: Some observations on track autoradiographs of biological specimens. Biochim. biophys. Acta **7** (1951) 198. — ⟨142⟩ —.

[262] LEVI, H.: Improved α-track autoradiographs of biologic specimens. Nature **171** (1953) 123. — ⟨142⟩ —.

[263] LEVI, H.: Quantitative β-track autoradiography of single cells. Exp. Cell Res. **7** (1954) 44. — ⟨143⟩ —.

[264] LEVI, H.: A discussion of recent advances towards quantitative autoradiography. Exp. Cell Res. **13** Suppl. 4 (1957) 207. — ⟨143⟩ —.

[265] LEVI, H. and A. S. HOGBEN: Quantitative β-track autoradiography with nuclear track emulsions. Kong. danske Vidensk. Selsk. mat.-fysiske Medd. **30** (1955) No. 1. p. 1. — ⟨143⟩ —.

[266] LEVI, H. and A. NIELSEN: Quantitative evaluation of autoradiograms on the basis of track or grain counting. Lab. Invest. **8** (1959) 82. — ⟨143⟩ —.

[267] LEVI, H., A. W. ROGERS, M. WEIS BENTZON and A. NIELSEN: On the quantitative evaluation of autoradiograms. Kong. danske Vidensk. Selsk. mat.-fysiske Medd. **33** (1963) No. 11, 1. — ⟨143⟩ —.

[268] LIBBY, R. L.: The use of tagged antigens in immunochemical studies. Trans. N. Y. Acad. Sci. **9** (1947) 248. — ⟨42⟩ —.

[269] LINDENBAUM, A. and R. E. ALPER: Electron microscopic autoradiography of alpha particles and protons. Atompraxis **12** (1966) 127. — ⟨104⟩ —.

[270] LIQUIER-MILWARD, J.: Track-radioautographic study of intracellular localization of cobalt in neoplastic tissues. Biochim. biophys. Acta **14** (1954) 459. — ⟨142⟩ —.

[271] LIQUIER-MILWARD, J.: Electron microscopy and radioautography as coupled techniques in tracer experiments. Nature **177** (1956) 619. — ⟨91, 102, 132⟩ —.

[272] LLOYD, E., J. H. MARSHALL, J. W. BUTLER and R. E. ROWLAND: A computer programme for automatic scanning of autoradiographs and micrographs of bone sections. Nature **211** (1966) 663. — ⟨144⟩ —.

[273] LONGINOV, M. F.: Quantitative evaluation of dentritic segregation in steel through autoradiography without the use of standards. Nucl. Sci. Abstr. **14** (1960) Abstr. No. 19357; "Metallurgy and Metallography," p. 387—392. — ⟨159⟩ —.

[274] LOTZ, W. E., J. C. GALLIMORE and G. A. BOYD: How to get good gross autoradiographs of large undecalcified bones. Nucleonics **10** (1952) 28. — ⟨41⟩ —.

[275] LÜTHI, U. and P. G. WASER: Low-temperature fluorography induced by tritium-labelled compounds on thin-layer chromatograms. Nature **205** (1965) 1190. — ⟨27⟩ —.

[276] LÜTHI, U. and P. G. WASER: Thin-layer fluorography of tritium-labelled compounds. Adv. Teac. Meth. **3** (1966) 149 and Atomlight **50** (1966). — ⟨27⟩ —.

[277] LUPULESCU, A. and A. PETROVICI: Étude radio-autographique en microscopie électronique de l'I^{131} dans la thyroïde du rat. Arch. Anat. micr. Morph. exp. **54** (1965) 895. — ⟨132⟩ —.

[278] LUPULESCU, A. and A. PETROVICI: Electron microscopic autoradiography of radioiodine (^{131}I) in the thyroid gland. Acta biol. med. germ. **16** (1966) 86. — ⟨132⟩ —.

[279] MACDONALD, A. M., J. COBBS, A. K. SOLOMON and D. STEINBERG: Stripping film technic for radioautographs. Proc. Soc. exp. Biol. (N. Y.) **72** (1949) 117. — ⟨61⟩ —.

[280] MAKIN, S. M.: The use of irradiated extraction replicas to identify inclusions and precipitates in metals: a preliminary note. Int. J. appl. Radiat. **7** (1960) 258. — ⟨21, 22⟩ —.

[281] MAKIN, S. M. and A. E. NUNLEY: An autoradiographic method for determining the distribution of iron on recording tape. Int. J. appl. Radiat. **7** (1959) 123. — ⟨50, 51⟩ —.

[282] MALMON, A. G.: Electron microscope observation of fission fragment tracks in plastic. J. appl. Physics **34** (1963) 3634. — ⟨122⟩ —.

[283] MALMON, A. G.: Fission fragment tracks as uranium tracers in biological. electron microscopy. Biophys. J. **4** (1964) 1. — ⟨122⟩ —.

[284] MALMON, A. G.: High resolution isotope tracing in electron microscopy using induced nuclear reactions. J. theor. Biol. **9** (1965) 77. — ⟨123⟩ —.

[285] MAMUL, YA. V.: Quantitative autoradiography using a radioactive wedge. Int. J. appl. Radiat. **1** (1956) 178. — ⟨152⟩ —.

[286] MAMUL, YA. V.: Post mortem diffusion of tissue substances as a source of artefacts in autoradiography. (Russian.) Biofizika (Moskva) **4** (1959) 119. — ⟨81⟩ —.

[287] MANGOLD, H. K., R. KAMMERECK and D. C. MALINS: Thin-layer chomatography as an analytical and preparative tool in lipid radiochemistry. Microchem. J., Sympos. Vol. II (1962) 697. — ⟨26⟩ —.

[288] MARALDI, N. M. and B. DI CATERINO: Simple devices for preparing monolayers of nuclear emulsions in electron microscopy autoradiography. Sci. Tools (Stockholm) **15** (1968) 34. — ⟨111⟩ —.

[289] MARKMAN, B.: Autoradiography of tritium chromatograms. J. Chromatogr. **11** (1963) 118. — ⟨24, 25⟩ —.

[290] MARSHALL, J. H. and M. P. FINKEL: Autoradiographic dosimetry of mouse bone containing Ca^{45}, Sr^{90}, and Ra^{226}. II. The sensitive region in the induction of osteogenic sarcomas. Nucl. Sci. Abstr. **15** (1961) Abstr. No. 8515. — ⟨161⟩ —.

[291] MARSHALL, J. H., V. K. WHITE and J. COHEN: Microscopic metabolism of Ca in bone. I. Three-dimensional deposition of Ca-45 in canine osteons. Radiat. Res. **10** (1959) 197. — ⟨40⟩ —.

[292] MARSHALL, J. H., R. E. ROWLAND and J. JOWSEY: Microscopic metabolism of Ca in bone. II. Quantitative autoradiography. Radiat. Res. **10** (1959) 213. — ⟨40⟩ —.

[293] MARSHALL, J. H., J. JOWSEY and R. E. ROWLAND: Microscopic metabolism of Ca in bone. IV. Ca^{45} deposition and growth rate in canine osteons. Radiat. Res. **10** (1959) 243. — ⟨40, 161⟩ —.

[294] MARSHALL, J. H., R. E. ROWLAND and J. JOWSEY: Microscopic metabolism of Ca in bone. V. The paradox of diffuse activity and long-term exchange. Radiat. Res. **10** (1959) 258. — ⟨40⟩ —.

[295] MARTON, L. and P. H. ABELSON: Tracer Micrography. Science **106** (1947) 69. — ⟨119⟩ —.

[296] MASSAGLIA, A., U. ROSA and S. SOSI: Thin-layer chromatography of some ^{131}I and ^{125}I labelled iodopyrimidines and related nucleosides. J. Chromatogr. (Amst.) **17** (1965) 316. — ⟨28⟩ —.

[297] MAUNSBACH, B. and S. ULLBERG: Electron microscopic autoradiography of radioiodine in the thyroid using the extranuclear electron of J-125. J. Ultrastruct. Res. **7** (1962) 339. — ⟨132⟩ —.

[298] MAURER, W. and E. PRIMBSCH: Größe der β-Selbstabsorption bei der ^{3}H-Autoradiographie. Exp. Cell Res. **33** (1964) 8. — ⟨71, 153, 154⟩ —.

[299] MAZIA, D. and N. L. BUCHER: A method for avoidance of electrostatic flashing in preparing autoradiographs with stripping film. Experientia **16** (1960) 215. — ⟨63⟩ —.

[300] MAZIA, D., W. S. PLAUT and G. W. ELLIS: A method for quantitative assessment of autoradiographs. Exp. Cell Res. **9** (1955) 305. — ⟨147, 148⟩ —.

[301] McCOY, H. E.: Oxidation of beryllium in CO_2 by autoradiographic techniques. J. nuclear Mater. **15** (1965) 249. — ⟨19, 20⟩ —.

[302] MEEK, G. A. and M. J. MOSES: Localization of tritiated thymidine in HeLa cells by electron autoradiography. J. roy. micr. Soc. **81** (1963) 187. — ⟨106, 135⟩ —.

[303] MEEK, G. A., M. J. MOSES and A. EIRING: Abstract in: 1st Congress Am. Soc. for Cell Biology 1961, p. 140. — ⟨104, 106⟩ —.

[304] MÉREI, F. T. and F. GALLYAS: Quantitative determination of ^{35}S-methionine incorporated into proteins of cell groups or nuclei of the CNS. J. Neurochem. (Oxford) **11** (1964) 251. — ⟨161⟩ —.

[305] MESSIER, B. and C. P. LEBLOND: Preparation of coated radioautographs by dipping section in fluid emulsion. Proc. Soc. exp. Biol. (N. Y.) **96** (1957) 7. — ⟨76, 111⟩ —.

[306] MICOU, J. and L. GOLDSTEIN: A simple method to reduce the strain in manual grain counting of autoradiographs. Stain Technol. **34** (1959) 347. — ⟨142⟩ —.

[307] MILLER, B. F. and F. HOECKER: Quantitation of alpha-emitters in bone. Nucleonics 8/5 (1951) 44. — ⟨143⟩ —.

[308] MILLMANN, S. and L. S. FOSTER: Nucleonics applications, metallurgical applications of autoradiography. I. A literature survey. II. Preliminary experiments. Nucl. Sci. Abstr. **7** (1953) Abstr. No. 155. — ⟨10⟩ —.

[309] MIZUHIRA, V.: Electron-microscopic autoradiography on domestic fresh photographic emulsions and developing methods, for nucleus studies. Radioisotopes (Tokyo) **14** (1965) 240 (Japan.) and in: Nucl. Sci. Abstr. **20** (1966) Abstr. No. 37050. — ⟨120⟩ —.

[310] MIZUHIRA, V. and K. UCHIDA: High resolution electron microscopic autoradiography. J. Histochem. Cytochem. **14** (1966) 765. — ⟨120⟩ —.

[311] MORICARD, R. and S. GOTHIE: Autoradiography in electron microscopy. Use of ^{35}S and ^{3}H. J. Physiol. (Paris) **55** (1963) 171. (French.) — ⟨132⟩ —.

[312] MOSER, L.: Über den Prozeß des Sehens und die Wirkung des Lichts auf alle Körper. Poggendorf Ann. **56** (1842) 177. — ⟨14⟩ —.

[313] MOSES, M. J.: Application of autoradiography to electron microscopy. J. Histochem. Cytochem. **12** (1964) 115. — ⟨105⟩ —.

[314] MOSES, V. and K. K. LONBERG-HOLM: A semiautomatic device for measuring radioactivity on two-dimensional paper chromatograms. Analyt. Biochem. **5** (1963) 11. — ⟨23⟩ —.

[315] MYERS, H. M., E. JENNINGS and H. BECKS: A rapid radioautographic technic for combined calcified and soft tissues. J. dent. Res. **31** (1952) 416. — ⟨38⟩ —.

[316] NADLER, N. J.: Measurement of the rate of iodine incorporation into the colloid of thyroid follicles by quantitative radioautography. J. Histochem. Cytochem. **1** (1953) 377 (Abstract). — ⟨161⟩ —.

[317] NAKAI, T.: Study of the ultrastructural localization of hair creatin synthesis utilizing electron microscopic autoradiography in a magnetic field. J. Cell Biol. **21** (1964) 63. — ⟨120, 121, 137⟩ —.

[318] NAKAYAMA, K.: Diagnostic significance of radioactive isotopes in early cancer of the alimentary tract, especially the esophagus and the cardia. Surgery **39** (1956) 736. — ⟨59⟩ —.

[319] Narath, A. and D. Gundlach: Quantitative Autoradiographie tritierter Verbindungen in Papierchromatogrammen. Angew. Chem. **72** (1960) 707. — ⟨159⟩ —.

[320] Neumann, D.: Technik der elektronenoptischen Autoradiographie in der Biologie, Part I: Acta histochem. (Jena) **33** (1969) 191; Part II: ibid. 217. — ⟨91⟩ —.

[321] New England Nuclear Corp. — Firm prospectus, 27 M-369-TM 200. — ⟨27⟩—.

[322] Neskovic, B. A.: A possibility of the application of quantitative autoradiohistography in detection of iodine J-131 in the thyroid. Acta med. jugosl. **15** (1961) 488 (French.). — ⟨161⟩ —.

[323] Noggle, T. S. and J. O. Stiegler: Electron microscope observations of fission fragment tracks in thin films of UO_2. J. appl. Physics **31** (1960) 2199. — ⟨122⟩ —.

[324] Norris, W. P. and P. E. Jenkins: Epoxy resin embedding in contrast radioautography of bones and teeth. Stain Technol. **35** (1960) 253. — ⟨38⟩ —.

[325] O'Brien, R. T. and L. A. George, II: Preparation of autoradiograms for electron microscopy. Nature **183** (1959) 1461. — ⟨104, 106, 132⟩ —.

[326] Odeblad, E.: Contribution to the theory and technique of quantitative autoradiography. Acta radiol. (Suppl.) **93** (1952) 88. — ⟨140⟩ —.

[327] Odeblad, E.: Matrix theory of quantitative apposition autoradiography. Acta radiol. **45** (1956) 324. — ⟨140⟩ —.

[328] Odeblad, E.: Further approximate studies on beta ray absorption and transmission. Acta radiol. **48** (1957) 289. — ⟨152⟩ —.

[329] Odeblad, E.: Matrix theory for quantitative evaluation of autoradiographs. Lab. Invest. 8 (1959) 113. — ⟨140⟩ —.

[330] Oehlert, W.: Autoradiographische Untersuchungen zur physiologischen Regeneration und Kanzerisierung. Acta histochem. (Jena) Suppl. VIII (1968) 257. — ⟨161⟩ —.

[331] Ostrowski, K. and E. A. Barnard: Application of isotopically-labelled specific inhibitors as a method in enzyme cytochemistry. Exp. Cell Res. **25** (1961) 465. — ⟨50⟩ —.

[332] Ostrowski, K., E. A. Barnard, Z. Stocka and Z. Darzynkiewicz, Z.: Autoradiographic methods in enzyme cytochemistry. I. Localization of acetylcholinesterase activity using a tritiated labelled irreversible inhibitor. Exp. Cell Res. **31** (1963) 89. — ⟨50⟩ —.

[333] Ostrowski, K., E. A. Barnard, Z. Darzynkiewicz and D. Rymaszewska: Autoradiographic methods in enzyme cytochemistry. III. Measurements on esterases in the cells of mouse kidney. Exp. Cell. Res. **36** (1964) 43. — ⟨50⟩ —.

[334] Otero-Vilardebo, L., N. Lane and G. C. Godman: Some characteristics of cells secreting sulfated mucopolysaccharides. J. Histochem. Cytochem. **12** (1964) 34. — ⟨135⟩ —.

[335] Ottendorfer, L. J. and H. Weisz: Semiquantitative Autoradiographie mit Hilfe des Ringofens. II. Genauigkeit und Empfindlichkeit. Mikrochim. Acta (Wien) **1962**, 725. — ⟨160⟩ —.

[336] Painter, R. B. and R. M. Drew: Studies on deoxyribonucleic acid metabolism in human cancer cell cultures (HeLa). I. The temporal relationships of DNA synthesis to mitosis and turnover time. Lab. Invest. 8 (1959) 278. — ⟨162⟩ —.

[337] La Palme, J. and P. Demers: Regression of the latent image of nuclear tracks in the photographic emulsion. Physic. Rev. **72** (1947) 536. — ⟨124⟩ —.

[338] PATTERSON, R.: Use of I^{131} labelled antigens in gel diffusion precipitate reactions. J. Lab. Clin. Med. **57** (1961) 657. — ⟨32⟩ —.

[339] PATZSCHKE, K.: Ganztier-Autoradiographie (Eine Methode in der Arzneimittelforschung). Münch. med. Wschr. **36** (1968) 2043. — ⟨46⟩ —.

[340] PAWELETZ, N.: Präparationsmethoden für die elektronenmikroskopische Autoradiographie. Firm of Siemens, (Special publication Eg. 1/201. June 1967). — ⟨106, 108⟩ —.

[341] PEARSE, A. G. E.: Localization of dehydrogenase and diaphorase systems with monotetrazolium salts and metal chelation. Biochem. J. **68** (1958) 17 P. — ⟨160⟩ —.

[342] PELC, S. R.: Autoradiograph technique. Nature **160** (1947) 749. — ⟨61⟩ —.

[343] PELC, S. R.: The stripping-film technique of autoradiography. Int. J. appl. Radiat. **1** (1956) 172. — ⟨33⟩ —.

[344] PELC, S. R.: Quantitative aspects of autoradiography. Exp. Cell Res. Suppl. **4** (1957) 231. — ⟨61, 149⟩ —.

[345] PELC, S. R.: On the question of automatic or visual grain counting. Lab. Invest. **8** (1959) 127. — ⟨142⟩ —.

[346] PELC, S. R.: Theory of electron autoradiography. J. roy. micr. Soc. **81** (1963) 131. — ⟨92, 94, 96, 97⟩ — .

[347] PELC, S. R., J. D. COOMBES and G. C. BUDD: On the adaptation of autoradiographic techniques for use with the electron microscope. Exp. Cell Res. **24** (1961) 192. — ⟨97, 103, 104, 132⟩ — .

[348] PERLMANN, P. and T. HULTIN: Autoradiographic analysis on agar plates of labelled antigens from rat liver. Nature **182** (1958) 1530. — ⟨33⟩ —.

[349] PERRY, R. P.: Quantitative Autoradiography. In: "Methods in Cell Physiology" Vol. I, p. 304—326, Academic Press. Inc., New York 1964. — ⟨154⟩ —.

[350] PILGRIM, C. and W. MAURER: Autoradiographische Bestimmung der DNS-Verdopplungszeit verschiedener Zellarten von Maus und Ratte bei Doppelmarkierung mit ^{3}H- und ^{14}C-Thymidin. Naturwissenschaften **49** (1962) 544. — ⟨162⟩ —.

[351] PILGRIM C. and W. MAURER: Autoradiographische Untersuchungen über die Konstanz der DNS-Verdopplungs-Dauer bei Zellarten von Maus und Ratte durch Doppelmarkierung mit ^{3}H- und ^{14}C-Thymidin. Exp. Cell Res. **37** (1965) 183. — ⟨162⟩ —.

[352] PILGRIM, C., K. J. LENNARTZ, K. WEGENER, S. HOLLWEGE and W. MAURER: Autoradiographische Untersuchungen über tageszeitliche Schwankungen des H-3-Index und des Mitose-Index bei Zellarten der ausgewachsenen Maus, des Rattenfetus sowie bei Ascites-Tumorzellen. Z. Zellforsch. **68** (1965) 138. — ⟨163⟩ —.

[353] PREUSS, L. E. and D. L. JOFTES: Autoradiography: Terminology and Definition (Letter). Science **126** (1957/II) 369. — ⟨1⟩ —.

[354] PRZYBYLSKI, R. J.: Electron microscope autoradiography. Exp. Cell Res. **24** (1961) 181. — ⟨111, 121, 128, 134⟩ —.

[355] QUASTLER, H. and F. G. SHERMAN: Cell population kinetics in the intestinal epithelium of the mouse. Exp. Cell res. **17** (1959) 420. — ⟨162⟩ —.

[356] RABINOWICZ, E.: Autoradiography of metal surfaces using a radiochemical method. Nature **170** (1952) 1029. — ⟨14⟩ —.

[357] RADEBRECHT, H. J. and S. BINNEWIES: Quantitative Autoradiographie von markierten Verbindungen in Papier-Chromatogrammen. Clin. chim. Acta **7** (1962) 873. — ⟨159⟩ —.

[358] RADWAN, M.: Anwendung der Autoradiographie zur Untersuchung der Struktur von Legierungen. Isotopentechnik **2** (1962) 270. — ⟨12, 14⟩ —.

[359] RAY, R. C. and G. W. W. STEVENS: Reciprocity failure and latent-image fading in autoradiography. Brit. J. Radiol. **26** (1953) 362. — ⟨124⟩ —.

[360] REINHOLZ, E., V. BELLOCH-ZIMMERMANN and CH. WIRTH: Zur Methodik der Gefrierschnitt-Mikroautoradiographie. Experientia **16** (1960) 286. — ⟨142⟩ —.

[361] REITH, A., B. SCHÜLER, W. VOGELL and M. KLINGENBERG: Elektronenmikroskopisch-autoradiographische Untersuchungen zur intramitochondrialen Lokalisation ^{3}H-markierter Adeninnucleotide. Histochemie **11** (1968) 33. — ⟨135⟩ —.

[362] REVEL, J. P. and HAY, E. D.: Autoradiographic localisation of DNA synthesis in a specific ultrastructural component of the interphase nucleus. Exp. Cell Res. **25** (1961) 474. ⟨106, 134, 135⟩.

[363] REVEL, J. P. and E. D. HAY: An autoradiographic and electron microscopic study of collagen synthesis in differentiating cartilage. Z. Zellforsch. **61** (1963) 110. — ⟨111, 128⟩ —.

[364] RICHARDSON, G. S., I. WELIKY, W. BATCHELDER, M. GRIFFITH and L. L. ENGEL: Radioautography of carbon-14 and tritium labelled steroids on thin-layer chromatograms. J. Chromatogr. **12** (1963) 115. — ⟨24, 26, 30⟩ —.

[365] RIEDEL, G.: Kernspurmikrofilme für die Elektronenmikroskopie. ZEISS-Informationen **15** (1967) 113. — ⟨117, 118⟩ —.

[366] RITZÉN, M., L. HAMMARSTRÖM and S. ULLBERG: Autoradiographic distribution of 5-hydroxytryptamine and 5-hydroxytryptophan in the mouse. Biochem. Pharmacol. **14** (1965) 313. — ⟨47⟩ —.

[367] ROGERS, A. W.: Autoradiography of tritium-labelled compounds on paper chromatograms. Nature **184** (1959) 721. — ⟨24, 25⟩ —.

[368] ROGERS, A. W.: The rapid quantitation of silver grains in autoradiographs of tissue sections. J. Physiol. **152** (1960) 41 P. — ⟨145⟩ —.

[369] ROGERS, A. W.: A simple photometric device for the quantitation of silver grains in autoradiographs of tissue sections. Exp. Cell Res. **24** (1961) 228. — ⟨145⟩ —.

[370] ROGERS, A. W.: Die Mikroskopie von Autoradiographien. LEITZ-Mitt. Wiss. u. Techn. III/2 (1964) 43. — ⟨73, 74⟩ —.

[371] ROGERS, A. W.: The photometric measurement of grain densities in autoradiographs. J. Physiol. **190** (1967) 14 P. — ⟨145⟩ —.

[372] ROGERS, G. T. and D. E. GLANVILLE: Autoradiographic location of small amounts of chromium, manganese, and copper in aluminium-zinc-magnesium alloys. J. Inst. Metals **90** (1962) 354. — ⟨10⟩ —.

[373] ROGERS, G. T. and J. D. H. HUGHES: High resolution autoradiography of chemically reactive surfaces. Nature **199** (1963) 566. — ⟨16⟩ —.

[374] ROHR, H. P.: Die Kollagensynthese in ihrer Beziehung zur submikroskopischen Struktur des Osteoblasten (Elektronenmikroskopisch-autoradiographische Untersuchungen mit Tritium-markiertem Prolin). Virchows Arch. path. Anat. **338** (1965) 342. — ⟨135⟩ —.

[375] ROHR, H. P., W. KLIETMANN and W. OEHLERT: Durchführung und Anwendungsmöglichkeiten der elektronenmikroskopischen Autoradiographie. Z. ges. exp. Med. **139** (1965) 344. — ⟨115⟩ —.

[376] ROHR, H. P., J. SCHMALBECK and A. FELDHEGE: Elektronenmikroskopisch-autoradiographische Untersuchungen über die Eiweißsynthese in der Brunnschen Drüse der Maus. Z. Zellforsch. **80** (1967) 183. — ⟨135⟩ —.

[377] ROHR, H. P., S. WALTER and E. MAHRT: Die Mucopolysaccharidsynthese in ihrer Beziehung zur submikroskopischen Struktur der Knorpelzelle (Elektronenmikroskopisch-autoradiographische Untersuchungen mit Tritium-markierter Glukose). Verh. dtsch. Ges. Path. **49** (1965) 304. — ⟨135⟩ —.
[378] ROHR, H. P. and H. WENDT: Elektronenmikroskopisch-autoradiographische Untersuchungen zur Kollagensynthese der Fibroblasten in heilenden Hautwunden. Arch. klin. exp. Derm. **223** (1965) 605. — ⟨135⟩ —.
[379] ROHR, H. P. and H. U. ZOLLINGER: Die sogenannte „Zuckerspeicherniere" unter besonderer Berücksichtigung elektronenoptisch-autoradiographischer Untersuchungen mit 14-C-Saccharose. Virchows Arch. path. Anat. **341** (1966) 115. — ⟨135⟩ —.
[380] ROSENBAUM, E. H. and S. B. REICH: Binding of radiographic (I^{131}-labelled) contrast media to serum proteins demonstrated by immunoelectrophoresis and radioautography. Radiology **86** (1966) 515. — ⟨32⟩ —.
[381] ROSS, R. and E. P. BENDITT: Wound healing and collagen formation. I. Sequential changes in components of guinea pig skin wounds observed in the electron microscope. J. Biophys. Biochem. Cytol. **11** (1961) 177. — ⟨137⟩ —.
[382] ROSS, R. and E. P. BENDITT: Wound healing and collagen formation. III. A quantitative radioautographic study of the utilization of proline-H^3 in wounds from normal and scorbutic guinea pigs. Cell Biol. **15** (1962) 99. — ⟨137⟩ —.
[383] ROSS, R. and E. P. BENDITT: A comparison of the utilization of proline-H^3 in healing wounds as seen by electron-microscope autoradiography. Fed. Proc. **22** (1963) 190. — ⟨137⟩ —.
[384] ROSS, R. and E. P. BENDITT: Wound healing collagen formation. V. Quantitative electron microscope radioautographic observations of proline-H^3 utilization by fibroblasts. J. Cell Biol. **27** (1965) 83. — ⟨137⟩ —.
[385] ROTBLAT, J. and G. WARD: Analysis of the radioactive content of tissues by α-track autoradiography. Phys. in Med. Biol. **1** (1956) 57. — ⟨143⟩ —.
[386] ROWLAND, R. E., J. JOWSEY and J. H. MARSHALL: Microscopic metabolism of Ca in bone. III. Microradiographic measurements of mineral density. Radiat. Res. **10** (1959) 234. — ⟨40⟩ —.
[387] ROWLAND, R. E. and J. H. MARSHALL: Radium in human bone: The dose in microscopic volumes of bone. Radiat. Res. **11** (1959) 299. — ⟨40⟩ —.
[388] ROY, A. K. and O. W. NEUHAUS: Identification of rat urinary proteins by zone and immunoelectrophoresis. Proc. Soc. exp. Biol. (N. Y.) **121** (1966) 894. — ⟨31⟩ —.
[389] RUSSEL, W. J.: On the action exerted by certain metals and other substances on a photographic plate. Proc. Roy. Soc. (London) LXI (1897) 424. — ⟨15⟩ —.
[390] SALPETER, M. M.: Electron microscope autoradiography as a quantitative tool in enzyme cytochemistry. The distribution of acetylcholinesterase at motor end plates of a vertrebrate twitch muscle. J. Cell Biol. **32** (1967) 379. — ⟨158⟩ —.
[391] SALPETER, M. M. and L. BACHMANN: Autoradiography with the electron microscope. A procedure for improving resolution, sensitivity and contrast. J. Cell Biol. **22** (1964) 469. — ⟨100, 107, 111, 113, 124, 125, 131, 134⟩ —.
[392] SALPETER, M. M., L. BACHMANN and E. E. SALPETER: Resolution in electron microscopic radioautography. J. Cell Biol. **41** (1969) 1. — ⟨100⟩ —.
[393] SALPETER, M. M., A. ROGERS and E. BARNARD: Distribution of acetylcholinesterase at motor end plates evaluated quantitatively using electron

microscope autoradiography. Electron Microscopy and Cytochemistry Symp. Leiden 1966. — ⟨50⟩ —.

[394] Sawicki, W. and Z. Darzynkiewicz: Polyvinyl chloride protective films in autoradiography. Folia histochem. cytochem. (Kraków) **1** (1963) 283. — ⟨77⟩ —.

[395] Schaefer, H.: Nachweis und Messung kleinster α-Aktivitäten in biologischen Substanzen durch Bahnspurauszählung in der Photoemulsion. Strahlentherapie **77** (1948) 613. — ⟨143⟩ —.

[396] Schaefer, H.: Microtopologic coordination of histological α-ray radioautographs by means of a photocopy of the tissue structure. Strahlentherapie **94** (1954) 140. — ⟨89⟩ —.

[397] Schaefer, H. and A. Golden: Micro-alignment of alpha radioautographs by means of a contact replica of the tissue pattern printed with visible light. Exp. Cell Res. **5** (1953) 545. — ⟨89⟩ —.

[398] Schmidt, H. L. and G. Werner: Darstellung von ^{3}H-Atropin und ^{3}H-Nor(-)-Cocain. Liebigs Ann. Chem. **656** (1962) 149. — ⟨9⟩ —.

[399] Schneider, G. and W. Maurer: Autoradiographische Untersuchung über den Einbau von ^{3}H-Cytidin in die Kerne einiger Zellarten der Maus und über den Einfluß des Fixationsmittels auf die ^{3}H-Aktivität. Acta histochem. (Jena) **15** (1963) 171. — ⟨78⟩ —.

[400] Schneider, G. and G. Schneider: Über Stoffverluste bei Formol-Fixierung von menschlichem Gehirngewebe. Histochemie **4** (1964) 348. — ⟨78⟩ —.

[401] Schnünzel, G.: Über den Einsatz der Peltier-Kaskade für die histologische Gefriertrocknung. Acta histochem. (Jena) **30** (1968) 201. — ⟨35⟩ —.

[402] Schultze, B. and W. Maurer: Größe der RNS-Synthese in Nucleolus und Karyoplasma bei einigen Zellarten der Maus. Z. Zellforsch. **60** (1963) 387. — ⟨154⟩ —.

[403] Schwane, R. A. and R. S. Nakon: Radioautography and scanning of thin layer chromatograms of radioactive water-soluble substances. Analytic Chem. **37** (1965) 315. — ⟨27⟩ —.

[404] Seidel, H. S.: Cytostatika-Testung an individuellen Tumoren. Acta histochem. (Jena) Suppl. VIII, 1968. — ⟨161⟩ —.

[405] Selverstone, B., A. K. Solomon and W. H. Sweet: Localization of brain tumors by means of radioactive phosphorus. J. Amer. med. Ass. **140** (1949) 277. — ⟨59⟩ —.

[406] Shahon, D. B., N. B. Ackerman, A. S. McFee and D. W. Wangensteen: In vitro and in vivo radioautography in recognition and localization of gastric cancer. Proc. Soc. exp. Biol. **104** (1960) 350. — ⟨59⟩ —.

[407] Sheldon, H., J. M. McKenzie and D. van Nimwegan: Electron microscopic autoradiography. The localization of I-125 in suppressed and thyrotropin stimulated mouse thyroid gland. J. Cell Biol. **23** (1964) 200. — ⟨137⟩ —.

[408] Sheppard, H. and W. H. Tsien: Autoradiography of tritium-containing thin layer chromatograms. Analytic Chem. **35** (1963) 1992. — ⟨24⟩ —.

[409] Shiraishi, K. and R. Nagasaki: Behaviour of tritium in aluminium-lithium alloys. J. Nucl. Sci. Technol. (Tokyo) **2** (1965) 499 and Nucl. Sci Abstr. **20** (1966) Abstr. No. 19265. — ⟨16⟩ —.

[410] Shugar, D., A. Szenberg and H. Sierakowska: Exp. Cell Res. **13** (1957) 424. — ⟨160⟩ —.

[411] Siess, M. and G. Seybold: Über einen neuen Nachweis radioaktiver Stoffe in Gewebsschnitten durch Imprägnierung mit Silbersalzen. Klin. Wschr. **30** (1952) 601. — ⟨119⟩ —.

[412] SIESS, M. and G. SEYBOLD: Das Imprägnierungsverfahren der Autoradiographie von Gewebeschnitten. Z. wiss. Mikr. **63** (1957) 156. — ⟨119⟩ —.
[413] SILK, E. C. H. and R. S. BARNES: Examination of fission fragment tracks with an electron microscope. Phil. Mag. **4** (1959) 970. — ⟨122, 134⟩ —.
[414] SILK, M. H., A. O. HAWTREY, I. M. SPENCE and J. H. S. GEAR: A method for intracellular autoradiography in the electron microscope. J. biophys. biochem. Cytol. **10** (1961) 577. — ⟨118, 134⟩ —.
[415] SIMS, R. T.: The incorporation and fate of H^3-tyrosine in the hair cortex of rats observed by radioautography. J. Cell Biol. **22** (1964) 403. — ⟨137⟩ —.
[416] SJÖSTRAND, S. E., G. B. CASSANO and E. HANSSON: Distribution of sulfur-35 chlor-promazine in mice studied by whole body autoradiography. Arch. int. Pharmacodyn. **156** (1965) 34. — ⟨47⟩ —.
[417] SMITH, J. R. and H. A. FOZZARD: Localisation of tritiated "Digoxin" in the myocardial cells of frogs and dogs by autoradiography combined with electron microscopy. Nature **197** (1963) 562. — ⟨138⟩ —.
[418] SNYDER, F.: Quantitative radioassay methods for thin-layer chromatography: Zonal and autoradiographic scans (using H^3 plates, C^{14}, P^{32}, and I^{131} plates). Proc. Ser. IAEA, Vienna 1965, p. 531. — ⟨159⟩ —.
[419] SNYDER, F. and H. KIMBEL: An automatic zonal scraper and sample collector for radioassay of thin-layer chromatograms. Analyt. Biochem. **11** (1965) 510. — ⟨159⟩ —.
[420] SOGNNAES, R. F.: Preparation of thin "serial" ground sections of whole teeth and jaws and other highly calcified and brittle structures. Anat. Rec. **99** (1947) 133. — ⟨38⟩ —.
[421] SOGNNAES, R. F., J. H. SHAW, A. K. SOLOMON and E. HARVOLD: A method for radioautography of specimens composed of both hard and soft structures. Anat. Rec. **104** (1949) 319. — ⟨38, 39⟩ —.
[422] SPEH, K. C. and G. W. MORTON: Electronic scanner for neutron film badges. Paper presented before Amer. Phys. Soc. 30. January 1957. — ⟨143⟩ —.
[423] SPERLING, F.: Electron-track autoradiography of radioactive frog embryos. Nature **174** (1954) 749. — ⟨142⟩ —.
[424] STEIN, O. and J. GROSS: Electron microscopic autoradiography of the metabolism of iodine-125 in the thyroid gland. Exp. Cell Res. **31** (1963) 208. — ⟨137⟩ —.
[425] STEIN, O. and J. GROSS: Metabolism of iodine-125 in the thyroid gland studied with electron microscopic autoradiography. Endocrinology **75** (1964) 787. — ⟨137⟩ —.
[426] STEVENS, G. W. W.: Resolution testing in autoradiography. Nature **161** (1948) 432. — ⟨71, 91⟩ —.
[427] STEVENS, G. W. W.: Radioactive microphotographs for resolution testing in autoradiography. Brit. J. Radiol. **23** (1950) 723. — ⟨72, 91⟩ —.
[428] STILLSTRÖM, J.: Grain count corrections in autoradiography. Int. J. appl. Radiat. **14** (1963) 113. — ⟨154⟩ —.
[429] STILLSTRÖM, J.: Grain count corrections in autoradiography. II. Int. J. appl. Radiat. **16** (1965) 357. — ⟨154⟩ —.
[430] STÖCKER, E. and H. A. MÜLLER: Zur chemischen Induktion von Silberkörnern im Strippingfilm bei der Orcein-Quetsch-Technik. Histochemie **11** (1967) 167. — ⟨68, 69⟩ —.
[431] STOWELL, E. C.: Special-purpose slide rules as exemplified by a rule for maintaining a constant exposure in successive autoradiographs with iodine-131. Nature **198** (1963) 318. — ⟨157⟩ —.

[432] STUBBLEFIELD, E.: Quantitative tritium autoradiography of mammalian chromosomes. J. Cell Biol. **25** (1965) 137. — ⟨152⟩ —.

[433] STUMPF, W. E. and L. J. ROTH: Vacuum freeze drying of frozen sections for dry-mounting high resolution autoradiography. Stain Technol. **39** (1964) 219. — ⟨79⟩ —.

[434] STUMPF, W. E. and L. J. ROTH: High resolution autoradiography with dry-mounted, freeze-dried frozen sections. Comparative study of six methods using two diffusible compounds ^{3}H-Estradiol and ^{3}H-Mesobilirubinogen. J. Histochem. Cytochem. **14** (1966) 274. — ⟨79⟩ —.

[435] SÜSS, A.: Eine Methode zur autoradiographischen Untersuchung der Phosphorverteilung im Boden. Naturwissenschaften **46** (1959) 146. — ⟨57⟩ —.

[436] TAKEUCHI, T., M. SAKAGUCHI and Y. NAKAMOTO: Detection of latent fingerprint by autoradiography. Naturwissenschaften **45** (1958) 36. — ⟨52⟩ —.

[437] TAUGNER, R., H. HOLE, G. GRIGOLEIT and U. WAGEMANN: Herstellung geeigneter Gefrierschnitte zur Autoradiographie der Niere in einer Kühlkammer mit eingebautem Mikrotom. Naunyn-Schmiedebergs Arch. exp. Path. Pharmak. **234** (1958) 330. — ⟨35⟩ —.

[438] TAUGNER, R., P. SUPPLY, A. BRAUN, R. DROH and J. MAHN: Zur Gefrierschnitt-Autoradiographie am ganzen Tier. Nuclear-Medizin **3** (1963) 397. — ⟨35, 37⟩ —.

[439] TAUXE, W. N., A. H. MOSER and G. A. BOYD: Etymology of autoradiography. Science **120** (1954/II) 149. — ⟨1⟩ —.

[440] TER-POGOSSIAN, M., L. DONADIEU, G. MORENO and M. BESSIS: Effet d'un champ magnétique intense sur le rendement photographique en autoradiographie au microscope électronique. C. R. Acad. Sci. Paris **262** (1966) 2771. — ⟨120⟩ —.

[441] THURSTON, J. M. and D. L. JOFTES: Stains compatible with dipping radioautography. Stain Technol. **38** (1963) 231. — ⟨77⟩ —.

[442] TOLLES, W. E.: Methods of automatic quantitation of microautoradiographs. Lab. Invest. 8 (1959) 99. — ⟨144, 145⟩ —.

[443] TONNA, E. A.: On the distribution of reduced silver grains in autoradiograms of bone and cartilage following H-3-amino acid administration. Lab. Invest. **13** (1964) 1238. ⟨161⟩.

[444] TONNA, E. A. and E. P. CRONKITE: Factors which influence the latent image in autoradiography. Stain Technol. **33** (1958) 255. — ⟨124⟩ —.

[445] TUBBS, F. E., L. CREVASSE and M. W. WHEAT·jr.: Localization of tritiated digoxin in dog myocardium by electron microscopic autoradiography. Circulat. Res. **14** (1964) 236. — ⟨138⟩ —.

[446] VAN TUBERGEN, R. P.: The use of radioautography and electron microscope for the localization of tritium label in bacteria. J. biophys. biochem. Cytol. **9** (1961) 219. — ⟨132, 134⟩ —.

[447] TUDOR, S., A. WEISSTUCH and S. H. DAVANG: Application of autoradiographic techniques to battery research. Electrochem. Technol. **3** (1965) 90. — ⟨19⟩ —.

[448] TZSCHASCHEL, R.: Experimentelle Methoden zu einer quantitativen Autoradiographie in Mikrobiologie und Zellforschung. Atompraxis **4** (1958) 49 und 265. — ⟨152⟩ —.

[449] ULLBERG, S.: Autoradiography in general and points about its use in investigations with S^{35}-labelled penicillin. Acta radiol. Suppl. **118** (1954) 22. — ⟨37, 38, 47⟩ —.

[450] ULLBERG, S.: Autoradiographic distribution and excretion studies with S^{35}-labelled penicillin. Proc. Soc. exp. Biol. **85** (1954) 550. — ⟨47⟩ —.
[451] ULLBERG, S.: Autoradiographic studies on the distribution of labelled drugs in the body. Proc. Second. U. N. Int. Conf. Peaceful Uses Atomic Energy **24** (1958) 248 and Progr. Nucl. Energy (Biol.) **2** (1959) 29. — ⟨47⟩ —.
[452] ULLBERG, S.: Autoradiographic localization in the tissues of drugs and metabolites. Biochem. Pharmacol. **9** (1962) 29. — ⟨47⟩ —.
[453] ULLBERG, S. and G. BENGTSSON: Autoradiographic distribution studies with natural estrogens. Acta endocr. (Copenhagen) **43** (1963) 75. — ⟨47⟩ —.
[454] ULLBERG, S. and B. EWALDSSON: Distribution of radio-iodine studies by wholebody autoradiography. Acta radiol. **2** (1964) 24. — ⟨47⟩ —.
[455] ULLBERG, S. and W. KORANSKY: Autoradiographic investigation with slices through entire animals of the distribution of labelled substances. Naunyn-Schmiedebergs Arch. exp. Path. Pharmak. **246** (1963) 65. — ⟨47⟩ —.
[456] ULLBERG, S., A. NELSON, H. KRISTOFFERSON and A. ENGSTROM: Distribution of plutonium in mice; an autoradiographic study. Acta radiol. (Stockholm) **58** (1962) 459. — ⟨47, 48⟩ —.
[457] VINCENT, J., S. HAUMONT and J. ROLES: Microscopic determination of bone phosphorus by quantitative autoradiography of neutron-activated sections. J. Cell Biol. **24** (1965) 31. — ⟨161⟩ —.
[458] VINCENT, W. S.: P^{32} incorporation into starfish oocyte nucleoli. Biol. Bull. **107** (1954) 326. — ⟨78⟩ —.
[459] WADEWITZ, S. and A. MUELLER: The preparation of microautoradiographs with metallic specimens. Isotopentechnik **2** (1962) 81. — ⟨65⟩ —.
[460] WAINWRIGHT, W. W., E. C. ANDERSON, P. C. HAMMER and CH. A. LEHMAN: Simplified autoradiography exposure calculation. Nucleonics **12** (1954) 19. — ⟨156⟩ —.
[461] WALTERS, M. C. and R. THAINE: C^{14} β-track autoradiography of high resolution. Nature **173** (1954) 1146. — ⟨142⟩ —.
[462] WASER, P. G. and U. LÜTHI: Autoradiography of end-plates with carbon-14-calebash-curarine I and carbon-14-decamethonium. Nature **178** (1956) 981. — ⟨67⟩ —.
[463] WASER, P. G. and U. LÜTHI: Autoradiographische Lokalisation von ^{14}C-Calebassen-Curarin I und ^{14}C-Decamethonium in der motorischen Endplatte. Arch. internat. pharmacodyn. **112** (1957) 272. — ⟨66, 67⟩ —.
[464] WASER, P. G., U. LÜTHI and P. HUBER: Autoradiographischer Nachweis von ^{14}C-Calebassen-Curarin I und ^{14}C-Decamethonium in der Endplatte. Helv. physiol. pharmacol. Acta **14** (1956) 55. — ⟨67⟩ —.
[465] WEILL, R.: Recent achievements in dental histochemistry. Ann. Histochim. 8 (1964) 5 (French). — ⟨39, 44⟩ —.
[466] WEISZ, H.: Ein Trennungsgang in einem Tropfen. Ein Beitrag zur Ringofenmethode und Tüpfelanalyse. Mikrochim. Acta (Vienna) **1954** p. 376. — ⟨160⟩ —.
[467] WEISZ, H.: Anwendung des Ringofens in der Tüpfelkolorimetrie. Mikrochim. Acta (Vienna) **1954** p. 785. — ⟨160⟩ —.
[468] WEISZ, H. and D. KLOCKOW: On the temperature dependence of the "fading effect" in semiquantitative autoradiography by the ring-oven method (demonstrated with Ca^{45}, Tl^{204}, and Sr^{90}/Y^{90}). Analytica chim. Acta (Amst.) **33** (1965) 532 and 538. — ⟨124⟩ —.
[469] WEISZ, H. and D. KLOCKOW: Identification of radionuclides (e. g. Au^{198}) by semiquantitative radioautographic determination of their half-lives using

the ring-oven methods. Analytica chim. Acta (Amst.) **34** (1966) 456 (German). — ⟨160⟩ —.

[470] Weisz, H. and D. Klockow: Halbquantitative autoradiographische Bestimmung von ^{14}C-Aktivitäten im Pico- bis Nanocurie-Bereich mit Hilfe der Ringofenmethode. Analytica chim. Acta (Amst.) **37** (1967) 370. — ⟨160⟩ —.

[471] Weisz, H. and L. J. Ottendorfer: Semiquantitative Autoradiographie mit Hilfe des Ringofens. I. Allgemeines, Apparatur und Handhabung. Mikrochim. Acta **1961**, p. 191. — ⟨160⟩ —.

[472] Weisz, H. and L. J. Ottendorfer: Semiquantitative Autoradiographie mit Hilfe des Ringofens. III. Expositionsgerät mit kontinuierlicher Drehbewegung. Mikrochim. Acta **1962**, p. 818. — ⟨160⟩ —.

[473] Werner, G.: A method of the radioautogr. demonstr. of low-molecular water-soluble substances in tissue sections. 6. Int. Congr. Biochem. New York 1964, Abstr. V, p. 458. — ⟨79, 81⟩ —.

[474] Werner, G.: Eine autoradiographische Methode zur Darstellung nichtflüchtiger Stoffe in biologischem Material. 3. Int. Congr. Histochem. Cytochem. New York 1968, Abstr. p. 290. — ⟨79, 81⟩ —.

[475] Werner, G.: Stoffwechselanalyse und autoradiographische Darstellung von Atropin, Scopolamin (^{14}C, ^{3}H) und deren Metaboliten bei einigen Säugetieren. Radioakt. Isotope in Klin. Forsch. Vol. VIII (1968) 365. — ⟨79, 81⟩ —.

[476] Werner, G.: Ein Verfahren zur autoradiographischen Darstellung wasserlöslicher Substanzen in Organen und seine Anwendung in der neuropharmakologischen Forschung. Arzneimittel-Forsch. **19** (1969) 422. — ⟨79, 81⟩ —.

[477] Werner, G., P. G. Bosque and J. Carreres Quevedo: Autoradiographie et Fonction Rénale. C. R. Ass. Anat. **129** (1966) 1869. — ⟨79, 81⟩ —.

[478] Werner, G., P. G. Bosque and J. Carreres Quevedo: Autoradiographie et Morphologie Fonctionelle. C. R. Ass. Anat. **129** (1966) 1871. — ⟨79, 81⟩ —.

[479] Werner, G., P. G. Bosque and J. Carreres Quevedo: Radioautographische Untersuchungen mit Tritium-markierten Tropanalkaloiden. Abh. dtsch. Akad. Wiss. Berlin Kl. Chem. Geol. Biol. **3** (1966) 541 and 629. — ⟨79, 81⟩ —.

[480] Werner, G., P. G. Bosque and J. Carreres Quevedo: Radioautographische Untersuchungen mit polytop-markiertem ^{3}H-Atropin. Naunyn Schmiedebergs Arch. exp. Path. Pharmak. **253** (1966) 95. — ⟨79, 81⟩ —.

[481] Werner, G., H. Werner, P. G. Bosque and J. Carreres Quevedo: Eine Methode zur autoradiographischen Darstellung hydrophiler Substanzen in biologischem Material. Z. Naturforsch. **21b** (1966) 238. — ⟨35, 79, 81, 82, 83, 85, 86, 150⟩ —.

[482] Wilson, A. T.: Preparation of scintillation autographs. Nature **182** (1958) 524. — ⟨23⟩ —.

[483] Wilson, A. T.: Detection of tritium on paper chromatograms. Biochim. biophys. Acta (Amst.) **40** (1960) 522. — ⟨23, 24⟩ —.

[484] Wimber, D. E., H. Quastler, O. L. Stein and D. R. Wimber: Analysis of tritium incorporation into individual cells by autoradiography of squash preparations. J. Biophys. Biochem. Cytol. **8** (1960) 327. — ⟨71⟩ —.

[485] Wolfe, D. E., J. Axelrod and K. C. Richardson: Localization of norepinephrine in adrenic axons by light and electron microscopic autoradiography. 5th Intern. Congr. Electron Microscopy **2** (1962) 1. — ⟨138⟩ —.

[486] Wolfe, D. E., L. T. Potter, K. C. Richardson and J. Axelrod: Localizing tritiated norepinephrine in sympathetic axons by electron microscopic autoradiography. Science **138** (1962) 440. — ⟨138⟩ —.

[487] WOODRUFF, L. A. and W. P. NORRIS: Sectioning of undecalcified bone; with special reference to radioautographic applications. Stain Technol. **30** (1955) 179. — ⟨38⟩ —.

[488] YOUNG, B. A. and B. M. KOPRIWA: The use of the Gevaert NUC-307 nuclear emulsion for radioautography at the electron microscope level. J. Histochem. Cytochem. **12** (1964) 438. — ⟨100, 125⟩ —.

[489] ZEHENDER, F., W. HERRMANN and H. LEIBSSLE: Die Wirkung von Separatoren auf die Antimonwanderung in Bleibatterien. Electrochim. Acta **9** (1964) 55. — ⟨19⟩ —.

9.2. Reviews and monographs

i BASERGA, R. and D. MALAMUD: Autoradiography, Techniques and Application. In: Modern Methods in Experimental Pathology. Harper & Row Publishers, New York, Evanston and London 1969.

ii BOYD, G. A.: Autoradiography in Biology and Medicine. Academic Press Inc., New York 1955.

iii CARO, L.: Progress in High-Resolution Autoradiography. In: Biophysics and Molecular Biology **16**, p. 171—190. Pergamon Press, Oxford, London, Paris 1966.

iv HARBERS, E.: Autoradiographie als histochemisches Untersuchungsverfahren. In: GRAUMANN, W. and K.-H. NEUMANN: Handbuch der Histochemie, Band I, Teil 1, p. 400—598. Gustav Fischer Verlag, Stuttgart 1958.

v NIKLAS, A. and W. MAURER: Autoradiographie. In: Hoppe-Seyler/THIERFELDER: Handbuch der Physiologisch- u. Pathologisch-Chemischen Analyse, 10. Aufl., Band II, Teil 2, p. 734—773. Springer Verlag, Berlin—Göttingen—Heidelberg 1955.

vi OEHLERT, W.: Orthologie und Pathologie des Schwefelstoffwechsels der Zelle im Autoradiogramm. In: Handbuch der Allgemeinen Pathologie, Band 2, Teil 5/1, p. 671—696. Springer-Verlag, Berlin—Heidelberg—New York 1968.

vii REIMER, L.: Autoradiographie. In: Elektronenmikroskopische Untersuchungs- und Präparationsmethoden, 2. Aufl., p. 556—567. Springer-Verlag, Berlin—Heidelberg—New York 1967.

viii ROGERS, A. W.: Techniques of Autoradiography. Elsevier Publishing Company, Amsterdam, London, New York 1969.

ix ROTH, L. J. and W. E. STUMPF: Autoradiography of diffusible substances. Academic Press, New York, London 1969.

x SCHULTZE, B.: Die Orthologie und Pathologie des Nucleinsäure- u. Eiweißstoffwechsels der Zelle im Autoradiogramm. In: Handbuch der Allgemeinen Pathologie, Band 2, Teil 5/1, p. 466—670. Springer-Verlag, Berlin—Heidelberg—New York 1968.

xi SCHULTZE, B.: Autoradiography at the Cellular Level. In: POLLISTER, A.W.: Physical Techniques in Biological Research, 2nd Edition, Vol. III, Part B. Academic Press, New York, London 1969.

xii SJÖSTRAND, F. S.: Electron Microscopy Autoradiography. In: Electron Microscopy of Cells and Tissues, Vol. I, p. 413—435. Academic Press, New York, London 1967.

10. SUBJECT INDEX

Disc Electrophoresis

and Related Techniques of Polyacrylamide Gel Electrophoresis

by **Dr. rer. nat. H. Rainer Maurer**

Max-Planck-Institut für Virus-Forschung Tübingen, Germany

Second revised and expanded edition 1971
With 88 figures, 16 tables and 948 literature references. XVI, 224 pages
Bound DM 68,—; $ 19.75

This updated and revised monograph in English language brings together — as far as possible — the body of widely dispersed knowledge and experience obtained from methods in disc electrophoresis and related techniques of polyacrylamide gel electrophoresis. The book is intended to be a laboratory manual with the purpose od sparing the user time consuming literature study and technical errors as much as possible.
Included are exact procedures for the most varied separation problems, a survey of types of apparatus, descriptions of methods for detection and quantitation of proteins, nucleic acids, enzymes, antigens and radioactivities, a detailed treatment of micro disc electrophoresis, preparative polyacrylamide gel electrophoresis and many other techniques for special problems. In addition, this monograph also cites examples of results from research in biochemistry, clinical chemistry and food technology with the intention of offering suggestions and showing the versatility of the method. From the information in this book, the user should be able, without any previous experience, to solve his separation problems to his (her) satisfaction.

W DE G

Walter de Gruyter · Berlin · New York

Proceedings of the International Research Conference on Proteinase Inhibitors

Munich, November 1970

Consulting editors **H. Fritz, H. Tschesche**

Approx. XII, 304 pages. 1971. Bound DM 94,—, $ 28.00

Contents (extract)

Specific Isolation and Modification Methods for Proteinase Inhibitors and Proteinases (Affinity Chromatography);
Chemistry, Biochemistry and Structure of Proteinase Inhibitors from Animal Organs and Secretions, e. g. Human Serum, Colostrum, Bovine Organs, Pancrease, Submandibular Glands, Leeches-Isolation, Ascaris Lumbricoides and Protein. Chemistry and Biology of Proteinase Inhibitors from Soybeans, Lima Beans, Peanuts, Potatoes and Maize;
Studies on the Physiological Functions of these Inhibitors;
Theory of the Enzyme Inhibitor Interaction and Studies on Inhibitory;
Characteristics Structure of Basic Inhibitors of Bovine Organs and some Serine Proteinases (Trypsin, Chymotrypsin, Elastase, Subtilisin e. a.)

Walter de Gruyter · Berlin · New York

Hoppe-Seyler's Zeitschrift für Physiologische Chemie

Ed. by A. Butenandt, F. Lynen, G. Weitzel

with co-operation of K. Bernhard, H. Dannenberg, K. Decker, J. Engel, W. Grassmann, H. Hanson, H. Herken, B. Hess, N. Hilschmann, P. Karlson, E. Klenk, H. L. Kornberg, F. Leuthardt, R. Schlögl, G. Siebert, H. Simon, Hj. Staudinger, W. Stoffel, H. Tuppy, H. G. Zachau

Editors: A. Dillmann, G. Peters

1 vol. with 12 parts annually. Approx. 2300 pp. DM 420,—, $115.00

Zeitschrift für Klinische Chemie und Klinische Biochemie

Respons. Editor Joachim Brugsch, Ernst Schütte

Editor: Friedrich Körber

Ed. by Karl Bernhard, Heinz Breuer, Joachim Brugsch, Johannes Büttner, Hans Joachim Dulce, Günther Hillmann, Hermann Mattenheimer, Ernst Schütte, Dankwart Stamm, Hansjürgen Staudinger, Otto Wieland

With the co-operation of Klaus Borner, Eckehart Buddecke, Hans-Christoph Curtius, Manfred Doss, Hartmut Dost, Hans Faillard, Jörg Frei, Günter Fuchs, Erich Gladtke, Heinz-Werner Goedde, Erwin Hansert, Hans Ludwig Krüskemper, Georg Löffler, Kurt Oette, Ladislaus Róka, Ellen Schmidt, Gerhard Uhlenbruck

1 vol. in 6 parts annually. Approx. 1024 pp. DM 260,—, $71,25

W DE G

Walter de Gruyter · Berlin · New York

Bei Fragen zur Produktsicherheit wenden Sie sich bitte an:
If you have any questions regarding product safety,
please contact:

Walter de Gruyter GmbH
Genthiner Straße 13
10785 Berlin
productsafety@degruyterbrill.com